Guy Seaton

The Crisis in America's Nursing Homes

Published by:

Adverbage, Ltd.
New Ross,
Co. Wexford,
Republic of Ireland.

All rights reserved. No part of this book may be reproduced in any form or by any means without the prior written consent of the publisher, excepting brief quotes used in reviews.

First printing: January 2002. Printed in the United States of America.

ISBN 0-9541723-0-2

All rights reserved. No part of this publication may be reproduced or transmitted in any form or by any means, electronic or mechanical, including photocopy, recording or any information storage and retrieval system, without permission in writing from the publisher.

© Guy Seaton 2002

TABLE OF CONTENTS

ACKNOWLEDGEMENTS 5
PREFACE 7
INTRODUCTION: WHY IS THIS BOOK NECESSARY? 9
CHAPTER ONE: MEDICARE AND MEDICAID – HOW DO THEY WORK? 15
CHAPTER TWO: MY INTRODUCTION TO THE NURSING HOME INDUSTRY 33
CHAPTER THREE: THE HEALTHCARE ARMY 39
CHAPTER FOUR: THE LOOMING CRISIS 73
CHAPTER FIVE: 1973-1981 – INSPECTING AND ADMINISTRATING 113
CHAPTER SIX: SUBACUTE CARE AND THE NURSING HOME 119
CHAPTER SEVEN: GOING SOLO 131
CHAPTER EIGHT: WHEN THINGS GO BADLY WRONG 135
CHAPTER NINE: DEALING WITH DIFFERENCE 155
CHAPTER TEN: BEING THE BOSS 161
CHAPTER ELEVEN: ONWARD AND UPWARD 167
CHAPTER TWELVE: MAKING THE BEST OF IT 173

ACKNOWLEDGEMENTS

Over the years, I've had the honor of knowing an uncountable number of dedicated healthcare workers, including nursing assistants, cooks, housekeepers, janitors, administrative staff and professional associates. So many of these touch both my professional and personal life in significant ways that it's impossible to single anybody out. Thank you to you all. You've worked faithfully and with dedication for rewards in no way commensurate with your skills and level of responsibility.

The success that my healthcare facility, St. Luke's subacute hospital, has enjoyed could not have occurred without the input of Carmelita Dimaano, another nurse whose career has been devoted to the elderly. She and those like her cannot be thanked enough.

I would also like to acknowledge the help of my editor, Deirdre Nuttall, in bringing this project to fruition.

Without the many residents who entrusted their lives to the staff working under my direction, and without their families, this book would never have been started. The purpose of my leadership has always been to ensure that they received the best available care – they were never just bodies to fill beds, but real people who loved and were loved back.

Finally, and most importantly, thanks to Jackie, my wife of more than 25 years. Jackie is not just my wife and my friend – she is also a healthcare professional whose mission it has always been to ensure that her employees and residents are treated with dignity and respect. Her dedication and spirit have touched everyone she's cared for, and left the world a better place.

Guy.

PREFACE

My three decades in the nursing home industry have provided me with many opportunities for forming friendships, and for professional success – and also for disappointment, when I've been unable to provide the residents in my care with all they needed and with the caregivers they required. Although the past 30 years have witnessed momentous developments in medicine and in terms of life expectancy, the level of skill and funding made available to nursing facilities remains inadequate.

As I write, at the end of 2001, most of us are preoccupied by the dramatic and worrying events that are sweeping the world stage. That much is unsurprising. But we should not lose sight of the nation's elders, many of whom fought in the wars of earlier generations, and struggled to create the strong, successful country that America is today.

Those of us facing retirement now, or within the next twenty or thirty years, face an uncertain future. The standards of care that are considered acceptable in most nursing homes are already inadequate, and everything indicates that they will deteriorate in the years to come. In this book, I point to the problems that the industry, its residents and their families face today, the issues that we will have to deal with tomorrow, and ways in which we can make the best of the system as it stands, and work together to improve it. There are no easy answers to these problems – but ignoring the situation and allowing things to continue as they are will not make them go away or in any way alleviate the difficulties of those in care.

The nursing home industry is full of dedicated, caring individuals who are responsible for the welfare of our senior citizens. Sadly, they are often led by policy makers, investors and service providers whose only concern is to generate profits in a system of free enterprise. Now, profit-making is not a bad thing in itself, but the consequences of concentrating on profit in an environment with strict price controls and no restrictions on cost is a recipe for disaster, and one of the principal underlying factors behind the cases of abuse and neglect that occur in today's nursing homes. The easiest way to ensure profits is to cut costs, and this is what inevitably happens – at the expense of the quality of care giving.

We cannot assume that the caring staff in our nursing homes will dedicate their lives to caring for the elderly when all of the profits generated by nursing care facilities are diverted to investors, and little attention is given to increasing the quality of life of the residents, and the working conditions and pay of

The Crisis in America's Nursing Homes

healthcare workers. The latter need tools, knowledge and financial support to get the job done. We, the public, must demand that the taxes we pay go to support those who are truly in need. Or have we, as a society, already decided that the vulnerable elders who need our care do not deserve more than a bed, food and basic hygiene?

My 58 years have been a wonderful and challenging journey, both personally and professionally. I hope that my remaining years will be equally rewarding, and that I will be offered the opportunity to participate in the care of sick and disabled senior citizens, as I have so often in the past. My efforts have always been directed towards caring and supporting the elderly during their final years, and I am proud to affirm that the people for whom I have been responsible have been given the best care and attention possible, with the tools and employees allowed us. Another great source of pride is the fact that my leadership has allowed every nursing home I've cared for to strive towards, and reach, the highest standards set by the Joint Commission of Accreditation of Healthcare Facilities.

Guy Seaton.

California, January 2002.

INTRODUCTION: WHY IS THIS BOOK NECESSARY?

I wish that it were *not* necessary to write this book. Throughout many years in the nursing home industry, my professional goal has always been to provide some measure of improvement; to show guidance and leadership; to work towards improving the employees' work environment by making their labors meaningful to them; to develop programs and systems that will improve upon what went before. Because of circumstances beyond my control, my ongoing efforts have recently faltered, but I remain optimistic that we – the citizens of the United States – *can* provide the type of caregiving that will meet the medical, nursing and emotional needs of our elders, giving them the same care and attention that they gave to their children years before.

As things stand at present, most nursing homes have become no more than prisons for old people. Places to send our sick and dying so that they will be out of the way until their lives come to an end. Even though the windows do not have prison bars, and the doors are unlocked, the elderly residents are no less prisoners than are the inmates banished to prison camps and jails. We should be ashamed of ourselves. Our senior citizens are, quite simply, afraid to enter nursing homes because such institutions have become merely places to die, rather than in which to live.

All over America, nursing homes are run according to both federal and state rules and regulations. Most states have similar rules, and all enforce federal standards which are identical in each nursing facility. Although 66 percent of nursing homes are privately owned, 27 percent are non-profit organizations and 7 percent government agencies, they are all obliged to conform to identical criteria, removing individuality from the caring system. The homogenization of healthcare that has occurred during the course of the last three decades, has seen the living environment of facility-bound elders deteriorate and become increasingly abusive and neglectful. While many facilities do the best they can with the meager resources at their disposal, it becomes harder by the day. The best managed homes succeed in providing an adequate service by housing a mixture of Federal, state funded and private residents, thus increasing their income and the availability of capital to pay nursing and other staff. Sadly, these facilities are in a minority. Most will not or cannot provide the level of care that our mothers and fathers need.

The elderly may be weak, sick and even confused or demented, but they are *individual human beings*, with feelings, desires and needs. They deserve to be treated as honored members of our society. Instead, many find themselves living in tiny rooms, sharing their space with a roommate and surrounded by alien possessions instead of their own cherished belongings. They are often left in bed for between twelve and sixteen hours a day, because there are not enough evening and night shift nurses to care for them in a more active setting, and because it is easier for nursing staff to look after the bedridden.

In many nursing homes, rounds are only made twice a night, the first when the night staff begins work at 11 p.m., and the second just before the day shift arrives on duty. Night nurses routinely provide residents with a double layer of underpads and diapers so that they will not have to assist them in the washroom, making it necessary for the elderly people to soil themselves. The resident who goes to bed at 6 p.m. will stay there until 9 or 10 the next morning. The restless are restrained at night so that they will not injure themselves or fall from bed, and rails are installed on many beds simply to prevent their occupants from getting up to use the bathroom. Bed rails can prevent falls, but they also prompt frustrated patients to attempt to climb over them, exacerbating the possibility of serious injury.

Senior citizens in homes are rarely seen as individuals, as clients or guests of the facility. To the management, they simply represent beds that have been filled. They are seen as sources of revenue – to be blunt, they represent $120 a day. Every empty bed is a loss. Even lease payments and rental agreements are based on the number of beds in the home. How tragic it is that our society has come to think of senior citizens as mere occupiers of beds, rather than as people!

Why have things deteriorated so far? The answer is simple: money. We need money to pay nurses, rent, mortgages, equipment, bank-loans and more, and obtaining the proper reimbursement for expenses is an uphill battle. The problems of the elderly do not make for interesting news stories, and politicians always find more gripping banners to wave before elections. How much more exciting it is to talk of dramatic battles that must be fought overseas, of gang warfare or the death penalty than of the simple, unglamorous needs of the elderly!

I have worked in the nursing home business for over thirty years, as a caregiver, an inspector, a manager and an owner. It is painfully clear to me that the major factor contributing to the scandalous condition of nursing homes today is the level of staffing. The minimal level required by government is insufficient to provide the care and treatment that residents need. If our elderly parents required no more than a roof over their heads, and food on the table, nursing homes would provide an excellent service. But residents deserve much more than just basic care. Instead of looking after their charges, nursing managers, directors of nurses and charge nurses spend much of their time placating family members and residents, investigating complaints and trying to correct the problems that occur on a daily basis. They are left with little time in which to devise new programs which will improve the routine of nursing home life, and make the declining years of the residents full and happy ones.

I find myself forced to accept the sad conclusion that *no one* deserves to live or work in a nursing home under the conditions of the healthcare system of today. It is too easy for society to turn its back on the aged and put them in nursing homes, where they will be out of sight and, largely, out of mind. When families or friends complain to the nursing home, they are labeled as troublemakers or shunned by the system. When they appeal to enforcement agencies, these agencies simply use complaints as a justification for issuing citations and fines intended to show the public that state and federal government will not tolerate abuse and neglect in nursing institutions. If conditions are perceived to be completely unacceptable in a nursing home, it is closed. But closing homes is *not* the answer – there are already far too few to care for the ever-growing population of dependent elders. Issuing citations and fines is easy, but these measures do nothing to improve the situation. Changing management, increasing staffing levels, in-service education and funding – these are more responsible approaches to the problem.

The Crisis in America's Nursing Homes

The government recognizes that contemporary nursing homes are facing grave problems, but it will not acknowledge its part in causing them. Rather than addressing the issue of chronic underfunding, it has chosen to pass laws and regulations which increase the standards demanded of nursing homes, without increasing the funding made available to them. This inevitably augments the possibility of nursing homes facing citations, fines, and accusations of fraud. But *how* can standards be improved if funding is not made available? It goes without saying that true abuse, neglect and fraud must be eliminated. But today, supposed abuse, neglect and fraud are often created by the very regulations that exist to prevent them. The days of prohibition in the 1930s represent a parallel situation. The government created a crime, and then prosecuted all those who broke the new law! Effectively, the government made criminals of ordinary people doing ordinary things. Eventually, as we know, the situation became unsustainable and the laws were repealed. But government does not always learn from its mistakes. Increasing standards and compliance requirements alone will not solve the problems of nursing home abuse, neglect and fraud. Holding corporate ownership responsible for the actions of nurses' aides, licensed nurses and other professionals just doesn't make sense when these basic healthcare workers know that they are in dead-end jobs with no opportunity to advance professionally or financially. Where is their incentive to improve the quality of service they provide? Why should they give their all to a profession that returns so little? The government's bottom line seems to be to remove itself from the line of fire – to abdicate all responsibility for healthcare. If our leaders are serious about caring for the nation's most vulnerable members, they will federalize the nursing home system, placing federal government in charge of employees at all levels, thus providing them with a sense of unity and potential as well as secure benefits and the possibility to advance their careers. But it's too easy to leave healthcare in private hands, keep medical funding low and blame someone else when it all goes wrong. Sadly, the people who are hurt the most by leaving nursing care facilities in private ownership are the most vulnerable – the elderly residents whom the system should be protecting and serving. A corporation may go out of business, but it is not a human entity that feels pain or anguish. Privatization is not the key to every solution, especially in an environment in which price control prevails and at a time when a majority of Americans recognizes that the care of the elderly and the poor should be the responsibility of federal government. In America, airport security is usually managed privately – and the tragic fallout of this mistake is more than clear today. Our nation's love affair with a healthcare system set loose in a free-market economy has exceeded all reasonable limits.

As a people, we must now admit that our healthcare system has proven to be inadequate in providing for its citizens' needs. Those who suffer most from its shortcomings are the elderly, and most specifically, those among them who are no longer able to care for themselves. The levels of state funding for these patients – never high – have not risen at the same rate as inflation and the ever-increasing costs of medication and other essential healthcare items. Unless the decline in healthcare standards is addressed quickly, we will soon have a full-scale crisis on our hands.

Rather than dealing with the realities of a difficult situation, government authorities are restricting nursing homes' freedom in administrating their finances. To keep afloat, most homes offer care to Medicaid, Medicare and privately funded patients, creating a nightmare situation for administrators, who must account for every Medicaid or Medicare dollar spent, and prove that it has been used for Medicaid and Medicare patients, and only for them. Many homes have closed beneath the strain and others are barely managing to keep open.

Here, I offer my own experience as the private owner of a nursing home to illustrate how the state is failing both the carers and the cared for. I take an honest look at the current status quo, and make suggestions as to how we might work together to improve the system. And, not least, I offer practical advice on how to make the best of a bad situation. Throughout the book, the points I make are illustrated by case studies. *While these are all based on real-life situations, in most cases, names and places are fictional. Any resemblance to real people, living or dead, is coincidental.*

CHAPTER ONE:
MEDICARE AND MEDICAID –
HOW DO THEY WORK?

The United States of America is unusual in being one of the few developed, industrial nations that is not also a welfare state. American citizens are, by and large, responsible for their own health needs. Anyone who can afford to do so subscribes to a health insurance policy to cover his or her requirements in the event of becoming ill. Those who cannot are left to the untender mercies of an inadequate healthcare system.

The most vulnerable members of our society have limited healthcare options, and many – especially the elderly – depend upon Medicare and/or Medicaid, a health insurance system which has come under fire in recent years for its inadequacies in coping with the needs of an aging population. Of specific interest here is Medicare's failure to work effectively with the nursing homes that care for its beneficiaries. In short, the funding allotted to cater for these senior citizens is simply not enough to pay for the treatment and attention that they need. Nursing homes find themselves unable to pay for ideal staffing levels, and are held solely responsible when residents suffer as a result.

Investing in the old and the dying is not good business today. What do they have to offer the world? Their productive days are over, and it is time for the young. Rather than using our taxes to pay for their care, let's increase funding to homeland security, the space program and to pay for still more military industrial complexes! Why not increase politicians' salaries and keep taxes low? In the nursing home industry, resources seem sparser than ever, and still we keep hearing about how Medicare and other social programs are using up a huge percentage of our national budget. Where does all this money go? Not to the people who need it! Nurses and nurses' aides are the worst paid workers in the America of today. Even a bagger in a supermarket earns more than the certified nursing assistant whom we entrust to bathe, clean, assess and accompany our aged parents. For the wages he or she earns, we don't expect the supermarket bagger to carry our groceries home and put them in the refrigerator for us, but we demand that the nurses' aide put her – for it is usually a woman – heart and soul into caring for our elderly relatives.

The nursing home system that we have created for our elderly is inhumane; the capacity of human beings to harm others never ceases to amaze me. Our healthcare system has come to resemble a conveyor belt, rather than a holistic approach to treatment and assisted care. Most of us need to see a physician from time to time, and this is particularly true in the case of the elderly. According to most doctors' schedules, fifteen or twenty minutes are allotted to each patient, but on average, he or she spends only five minutes attending to them. The elderly who are in receipt of Medicare may have to wait for several weeks before getting an appointment. Medicare will not pay the doctor unless the visit is medically necessary for a specific disease and diagnosis – but healthcare issues are rarely that simple. If the doctor has to send samples to a laboratory for testing before making a diagnosis, he and the patient have a problem; Medicare does not pay for laboratory testing. The government's line is that, in order to save money, Medicare pays only for tests that it considers medically necessary for the diagnosis and treatment of the patient. It will not pay for screening tests – in other words, testing for diseases which may not be immediately obvious from the patient's symptoms. This means that it will only pay to test for diseases that are already evident, and not those that the doctor suspects of causing the problem!

If you are a Medicare recipient, and are admitted to an acute hospital, plans for your discharge are made from the outset. The hospital strives to move you out as quickly as possible, whether or not you are ready to leave. If home is not an option, other placement is sought. If you need skilled nursing help, you are directed to a local nursing home with a vacancy – not necessarily the one best suited to your needs, but the first one to take you, or one with which the discharge office has a personal and mutually beneficial relationship. Any time spent in investigating homes is time wasted. On admission to the home, you will probably lose contact with your personal physician, and be assigned to a house physician instead. You may have to wait for days before seeing the doctor, who is only paid for one visit a month. Regardless of his or her intentions, little time will be devoted to you and little or none to your family. The physician's only source of information about your needs is the nurse, and he or she will probably not update your treatment plan in any way.

And what are your living conditions like? You'll share a room with one, two, or three roommates. You'll have one chair, one bed, one nightstand and a small closet, in a total space of about eighty square feet. You'll share a toilet and a sink with three or more residents, and will have to use a communal bathroom at some distance from your room for bathing or showering. Once your room has been assigned to you, a nurses' aide will make an inventory of your personal effects, and introduce you to your roommate. During the next few days you will receive visits from the activity director, food services director and director of nursing – perhaps even the administrator. Soon you'll grow used to the routine that is common to nursing homes all across the nation. The wakeup call is at 6 or 7 in the morning, with breakfast arriving before you have been helped to get clean. You'll have about 15 minutes to eat breakfast, but as at lunch and dinnertime, you will have to eat what you're given without any say in the matter. After breakfast, you will be dressed and, if you are unable to walk, placed in a wheelchair or recliner. There you'll stay, sitting in the hallway outside your room, or perhaps inside your room watching television. Maybe you'll be placed in the activity room until lunchtime, where an activity such as bingo or handicrafts might be underway. If the weather is good, it's possible but unlikely that you'll be allowed outside in the afternoon. As the day progresses, nurses will bring you your medication and nurses' aides will drop by. Once a week or so, you'll be taken for a bath or shower in the common bathroom. You'll be taken there already in a state of undress, or, if you are lucky, wrapped in a sheet or bath blanket. It will be impossible for you to maintain a sense of dignity when you are dressed and fed. Most of the staff will endeavor to treat you professionally and helpfully, and ensure your privacy, but they just won't have enough time to do so. From early afternoon, staffing levels will drop and throughout the afternoon and evening there will be even less people to help you with your requirements. To make things easier for themselves, the staff will put you to bed before dinner, and that is where you'll eat. As soon as it's dark, the lights will be turned off. The night staff comes on duty at 11, and there are even fewer to care for you and the other residents. You may only see them as they begin and finish their shift. Leaving your bed to go to the bathroom will not be an option and you'll soon learn to rely on your diaper. Of course, you have a call bell, but if you use it too often, no one will answer it, or it will be turned off at the nurses' station. Even at the best of times, bells take 15 or 20 minutes to answer, so be prepared to wait.

Tomorrow will be exactly the same, and the day after, and the day after that ... if you are lucky, you won't develop bedsores, you will be kept clean and staff members will talk to you from time to time. If you're in one of the better homes you may even be able to pursue your interests to some extent, at least at the beginning of your stay. The quality of your life will not be measured in terms of pleasure, dignity or self-respect but according to the presence or absence of bedsores on your body. In good nursing homes you will be well kept – fed, washed and dressed. Your psychological needs will probably not be met, however, and your sense of self-dignity will be hard to preserve.

You have ceased to be a person; you have become a resident waiting to die or return to the hospital. There is no space – physical or emotional – in which you can be an individual.

The Background to Nursing Home Culture

In traditional – and especially rural – communities, the elderly were cared for in the home, as they still are in less urbanized societies around the world today. As industrialization grew throughout the nineteenth century, populations migrated to urban settings, and traditional family life changed. Much of this was for the better, but one side effect was the creation of a group of people classified today as "homeless" – indigent and elderly persons with a range of physical and mental health problems, and nobody to care for them.

By the end of the nineteenth century, towns and cities across America featured "boarding houses" which provided homes to those without families or a place to live. For a fixed daily or monthly rent, they supplied meals and lodging. As the boarders aged, however, they began to need more than just food and a place to sleep. They needed to be helped to dress, to eat and to keep themselves clean. Many even became chronically ill or disabled, and boarding house owners found themselves becoming amateur nurses. During the same period, tuberculosis was widespread, and there were many sanitariums caring for the ill. The mentally ill were also catered for in centralized sanitariums.

After the First World War – in around 1920 – state authorities began to be concerned about the public health standards of these boarding houses, and health and safety regulations were developed for boarding houses providing healthcare services. If they wanted to continue housing the disabled, they had to become licensed by the state to stay in business. Most, if not all boarding houses were managed by women who did the cooking, housekeeping and laundry services but who had not received any specific healthcare training. As states required new health standards – mainly for safety and space requirement – these boarding houses were replaced with small institutions usually containing 10 to 25 beds, which were modeled on nursing units in hospitals. Gradually, these institutions came to be known as "nursing homes". Some started to offer apartment living, while others provided care for the chronically ill and disabled. In the development of licensing regulation for the operation of nursing homes, which occurred in the first half of the twentieth century, the regulations that had been developed by the hospital system served as a model. This medical model still forms the basis of nursing home regulations today.

As the twentieth century progressed, pharmaceutical companies learned how to produce drugs to immunize against or cure many diseases. Surgical techniques also underwent great strides at this time. As a consequence of these developments, the life expectancy of Americans increased rapidly. More people survived to advanced ages, resulting in a greater number of people living for many years with disability or chronic illness. At the same time, there was a dramatic demographic shift from rural areas and small towns to cities, creating a situation whereby large numbers of elderly people were left without a family network to support them. The Great Depression of the 1930s had come and gone, and many of these elderly Americans had few savings and limited income. What was to be done? This was the environment that engendered Social Security and later Medicare and Medicaid, the American version of social healthcare for the elderly and the poor.

The debate about medical care for senior citizens began in the 1950s, at a time when the average life span was reckoned to be around 60 years old. Social security benefits today start at the age of 62 for reduced benefits, or 64 for full benefits, because it was thought during this period that the population over 64 would remain small and relatively inexpensive to maintain.

Medicare and Medicaid are, therefore, government programs that were designed to guarantee health insurance for the elderly and the poor. They were introduced during the presidency of Lyndon Johnson in 1965 as amendments to the Social Security act of 1935, and their implementation followed in 1966. Over the years, the various governments of the United States have endorsed different approaches to the system. For a time during the 1970s, it appeared that a healthcare system approaching the social welfare systems seen in many European countries and in Canada might be developed from the existing Medicare, but after Reagan came to power in the 1980s there was a general shift towards increasing privatization and corporate take-over of healthcare. This shift was not only practical, it was also philosophical, as the emphasis in nursing care moved from focusing on patients' needs towards striving towards an ever larger profit margin and investor contentment. One of the manifestations of this change was the move away from making Medicare payments according to the number of days patients spent in hospital, and the type of treatments they received, to diagnosis-based payments. Since 1983, Medicare's policy has been to make payments of fixed rates, according to the health problem with which the patient has been diagnosed. The theory is that hospitals cannot then overcharge for individual patients. The reality, of course, is that everyone is different, and not everyone responds in exactly the same way to the same treatment. Some patients, quite simply, require more time and attention than others. Ever since the 1980s, the primary goal of many hospitals and care facilities has been keeping costs to a minimum – reducing the length of hospital stays, keeping as many patients as possible out of hospital in the first place, and maintaining staff levels as low as possible.

Before 1987, a standardized set of criteria by which homes funded or partially funded by Medicare could be judged was lacking, and some unscrupulous nursing home owners took advantage of this situation to exploit their residents without offering them the quality care that they needed. In 1986, an important report by the Institute of Medicine revealed the abuse present in many homes, and, at last, minimum standards were agreed upon with guidelines including the limitation of the use of physical and chemical restraints and the obligation of the home to provide basic care. Fifteen years later, these basic standards are still not met in every healthcare facility.

Throughout the 1980s, and up until the present, approaches to medicine changed, as new technologies and treatments were patented and made available to an increasingly health-conscious public. Healthcare costs continued to rise in the 1990s, now at twice the rate of inflation[1], and federal healthcare reform was once more rejected by the Congress which saw socialized healthcare as communistic and in opposition to the American Way. By the end of this decade, 16% of the American population was left completely without healthcare insurance. Healthcare costs continue to rise in the new millennium, and are expected to do so throughout its first decade and beyond, with the numbers of uninsured also increasing. The current healthcare situation is generally perceived to be in a state of crisis. Many view Medicare to be unsustainable in its current form.

But How Does Medicare Function?

Medicare covers individuals aged 65 or older, and consists of two related plans, known as "A" – a hospital insurance plan – and "B" – a supplementary medical insurance plan. Plan A covers the larger part cost of hospital bills for up to 90 days for each period of illness. Care in a nursing home is paid for in total for the first 20 days if these follow a period of hospitalization, and in part for the following 80 days. Hospice care for the terminally ill is also covered. Repeated periods of hospitalization are paid for, so long as the patient has spent 60 consecutive days without treatment.

Plan B, Medicare's supplementary medical insurance plan, supplements the benefits that the hospital plan provides. It requires enrollment in a pay plan, and approved contributors are entitled to the payment of 80% of their physician and outpatient services by Medicare, as well as other health costs, including durable medical equipment and diagnostic tests.

---

[1] Information available from the PBS organization (www.pbs.org).

Clearly, one can use up all of one's "credits" under the Medicare system. When this occurs, Medicaid steps in. This is a health insurance program designed for people over the age of 65, who have already exhausted their Medicare benefits and who are unable to pay for healthcare privately, and for people under that age, whose income is low. Funding for the program comes from federal and state benefits, with all states required to offer Medicaid to citizens in receipt of public assistance. However, individual states can determine the criteria for admission to the program, which covers nursing facility care, home health services, family planning, diagnostic screening and other medical expenses.

Latterly, the increasing importance of managed care networks and health maintenance organizations, or HMOs, has further altered the implementation of Medicare policies. HMOs, as they are generally known, are groups that contract with medical facilities, physicians and employers to provide medical care to a group of individuals, usually paid for by an employer at a fixed price per patient. An important issue to bear in mind is that most HMOs are for-profit corporations, whose responsibilities to their stockholders take precedence over their responsibilities to their clients. The HMO has a high degree of control over the amount and type of healthcare that individuals receive – often, for example, one cannot continue seeing one's family practitioner, but must use the services of one of the physicians in the HMO's pay. Even if one *is* allowed to see one's regular doctor, he or she may only be able to provide a limited range of testing and treatment.

Supporters of HMOs claim that they bring affordable healthcare to a wider range of patients, while their detractors maintain that they cut costs by reducing the number of treatment options available, thus reducing patient choice. Many healthcare professionals and members of the public have beseeched government to regulate managed healthcare more closely, and give more rights to healthcare consumers. Two of the most contentious issues are the patient's inability to sue their health plan provider for malpractice, and whether HMOs should be obliged to pay for doctors' visits, or visits to emergency rooms, which occur outside the health plan's network. Unsurprisingly, health plans are resistant to regulation, maintaining that the inevitable legal battles would increase their overheads and ultimately the cost of providing healthcare coverage to the public. Many doctors and healthcare providers, however, feel that their ability to effectively treat and care for the sick people in their charge is negatively affected by the policies of health maintenance organizations, which veto certain forms of care and do not compensate medical and caring staff, effectively removing the variable of choice. Similarly, healthcare consumers are anxious to see their range of options expanded, allowing them to visit specialists outside their HMO's network.

Historically, the Democrat Party has tended to favor healthcare reform, while the Republican Party has resisted it. This has long been a difficult issue in congress, and as party divisions on the subject grow less distinct, a resolution seems as far away as ever.

Do HMOs work? They do what they were ultimately designed for: they provide reasonable coverage for the healthy, employed citizen, including preventative health and short-term treatment from family physicians. Unfortunately, they attempt to work together with Medicare, and fail. When the federal government decided to allow HMOs to expand into the Medicare market, various problems emerged. While HMOs provide higher rates for patients requiring treatment in a subacute care facility, their payments for subacute and ordinary nursing home patients alike are made later than Medicare or Medicaid payments. HMOs fail when it comes to providing coverage for patients with serious health issues. Persuading them to pay for specialist treatment is notoriously difficult, as their priority is, consistently, to reduce their costs, preventing their rates (at the time of writing, about $160 a month) from increasing, and maintaining a healthy profit margin. In order to do so, they limit the services available to their clients.

Medicare Today [2]

The Kaiser/Commonwealth 1997 survey of Medicare Beneficiaries, which included telephone interviews with 3,300 non-institutionalized Medicare enrollees, was carried out by Louis Har-

---

[2] An important source of data in this section has been the Commonwealth Fund and The Henry J. Kaiser Family Foundation jointly supported the Kaiser/Commonwealth 1997 Survey of Medicare Beneficiaries.

ris and Associates, Inc., from November 1996 through June 1997. The survey found a high percentage of Medicare beneficiaries to be at high risk of deprivation and associated health issues, with a substantial number (of both elderly persons and disabled persons of every age) living below the poverty line, and a strong correlation between low income and aggravated health problems. In fact, the lower the beneficiary's income level, the more likely he or she was to report difficulties in obtaining necessary services. Most Medicare beneficiaries were found to be in receipt of supplemental coverage – privately arranged in the case of the wealthier, Medicaid in the case of the poorer.

Today, Medicare finds itself in crisis. The percentage of the public in receipt of Medicare payments is growing as the population ages, and is expected to double within the next three decades. In 1999, Medicare cost the government 12% of the federal budget – twice the amount it cost twenty years before. This figure is set to increase dramatically, and economists and healthcare professionals are voicing grave concern about the problems that are certain to face the elderly and poor of tomorrow as well as the tax-paying population that will have to support them. There is no crowd-pleasing answer to the problem. Medicare needs more direct funding, and this will only be provided if revenue is redirected, if income taxes are raised, or if luxury items such as tobacco and alcohol bear a substantial national sales tax. None of these seem likely to occur in an administration led by President George W. Bush [3]:

WASHINGTON (Reuters) - Under pressure from states and health insurance firms, the Bush administration said on Thursday it had revised Clinton-era protections promised to millions of poor Medicaid patients using private health plans.

Democrats and patient advocacy groups said the new rules, which will be enforced within a year, favored the healthcare industry over patients' rights and weakened grievance and appeal procedures for people using Medicaid, the public health program for the poor and disabled.

---

[3] Reuters, July 16th.

Medicare and Medicaid – How do they Work?

Health and Services Secretary Tommy Thompson said the new rules gave states implementing Medicaid more flexibility and would replace the "excessive" rules signed by President Bill Clinton in his final days in office.

"The new proposed rules will ensure that states have the flexibility they need to protect patients while protecting the programs they may have already established," Thompson said in a statement announcing the new rules.

Patient advocacy group Families USA said the new rules watered down specific details on grievance and appeals procedures available to patients on Medicaid.

"Our concern is that they are not putting the Medicaid patients' interests first," said Joan Alker, associate director of government affairs for Families USA.

"These rules have significantly weakened the grievance procedures in favor of the managed care industry, which was the most important part of these regulations."

In terms of grievance procedures, the new rules grant health maintenance organizations (HMOs) more time to deal with complaints and states can in some cases set their own time frame.

For example, a patient's right of appeal in the case of emergencies has been changed from 72 hours to three working days, meaning if someone gets sick on a Friday they could wait until Tuesday before their problem is addressed.

Health department officials strongly rejected the claim that patients' rights were not being safeguarded and Thompson said the amended rules still guaranteed Medicaid beneficiaries the "timely right to appeal adverse coverage decisions".

In addition, he said Medicaid patients were guaranteed access to emergency room care, a second opinion when needed, direct access to women's healthcare services and other protections.

"This proposed rule ... gives states flexibility to implement these protections without jeopardizing Medicaid beneficiaries access to healthcare," said Thompson. He did not provide examples of what this "flexibility" would mean to states and how it would work in practice.

Under Clinton's plan, Medicaid regulations should have been in place by last April but were twice postponed by the new administration. Thompson said the new rules would now take effect next year.

25

"I want to have patient protections in place as quickly as possible. However, the previously issued rule went far beyond what Congress intended with the Balanced Budget Act and its excessive mandates actually threatened beneficiaries access to care under Medicaid," Thompson said.

Democrats have charged that by amending Clinton's rules, the Bush administration is undermining a compromise on Medicaid that was part of the agreement Congress reached in 1997 to balance the federal budget.

Under that arrangement, states could require Medicaid patients to join HMOs but, in exchange, the Department of Health and Human Services was asked to secure rights for Medicaid patients enrolled in those plans.

Health department officials said the Clinton rules were perceived by the states and health maintenance organizations as being "too burdensome and prescriptive," particularly when it came to the grievance procedure.

Three Democratic congressmen wrote a letter to Bush this week accusing the president of "retreating to the detriment of our most vulnerable citizens" by not implementing Clinton's Medicaid rules.

The Medicare crisis must be addressed before even more people fall victim to its inadequacies. In a recent survey, 75% of elderly or disabled New Yorkers reported that their premiums increased by $300 or more a year, and 67% said that they were finding it difficult to afford insurance, even cutting down on essentials such as food and medication to make payment. [4] Let's repeat that ... they are *cutting down on essentials such as food and medication to make payment*! Even in times of recession, this is a wealthy nation – but many of our elderly are suffering from malnutrition, because they can't afford to pay for both food and medication.

Another important area where Medicare falls short is in ensuring that its beneficiaries are in receipt of the specific medication they need. One-third lack prescription drug coverage, and these people, most of them elderly, are the most likely to take medication irregularly, or not to take it at all. As the demands on Medicare grow, so do the efforts of officials to limit spending as much as they can.

---

[4] Info Survey conducted by the Medicare Rights Center, and published on the Internet at <http://www.medicarerights.org>.

MEDICARE AND MEDICAID – HOW DO THEY WORK?

At the time of writing, Medicare provides health insurance coverage to one in seven Americans [5] – or perhaps one should say, "attempts to provide" as all the evidence points to its shortcomings in catering for an increasingly needy population. Sadly, it seems unlikely that congress will do anything to improve the situation, beyond continuing to pass laws intended to raising the standard of nursing care, without releasing the funding that would make these improvements possible.

Some Facts and Figures [6]

Most of the services provided by nursing facilities are funded, at least in part, by Medicare and Medicaid programs. Medicare long-term services fall into category A, as outlined above. These are associated with post-surgery or post-hospitalization care, including rehabilitation. Medicaid nursing facility services are provided to state residents considered to be eligible. According to recent surveys, there are almost seventeen thousand nursing facilities in the United States, with a total of almost two million nursing facility beds. 13% of these facilities are hospital based, while 52% form part of a chain and the remainder are individually owned and operated. 66% of nursing facilities are operated for profit and 27% not for profit. The government runs a meager 7%. On average, each facility employs fifty-three direct care staff, thirty-five certified nurses' assistants, eleven licensed practical nurses, and six registered nurses. 8% of residents are funded by Medicare, 68% by Medicaid and the remainder privately. Over one hundred thousand beds are reserved for patients with special needs, such as ventilator dependent patients, sufferers from Alzheimer's disease, or AIDS patients. 40% of Americans aged 65 and over will spend some time in a nursing home during the course of their lives, while about 5% of the elderly population (persons over 65) lives in a nursing home at any one time.

---

[5] Information from the Henry J. Kaiser Family Foundation.

[6] Data obtained by HCFA's Online Survey, Certification and Reporting Date (March 1997), HCFA's Medicaid Statistical Information System (MSIS) (1995), HCFA's Medicaid Data System (1995), US Bureau of the Census, Statistical Abstract of the United States (1996).

Medicaid patients account for more than one and a half million of the total number of nursing facility residents, and 69% of the nursing homes' costs and the average Medicaid payment per patient is around $90.00. An average of around $243 per day is paid for beneficiaries of Medicare – in other words, about 8% of the nursing homes' costs. Private and long-term care insurance pay the smallest portion, around 3%. Families and residents pay for 20% of the costs of nursing home care.

Medicare and private health insurance companies alike do not see the elderly dependants as clients who deserve service, but as factors that make costs increase and profits diminish. To deal with health insurance issues, the government has instigated two distinct organizational structures; the Health Standard and Quality contracts, which have state licensing offices to survey and enforce healthcare regulations and laws, and the Healthcare Finance Administration contracts, with fiscal intermediaries who reimburse for the services provided. These two organizations do not communicate with each other, as though their functions were not inter-linked. Before the system of reimbursement to nursing homes was changed, there were considerable incentives to improve services. Now, however, many homes are not equipped or staffed to care for the increasingly complex medical issues that they must cater for. The issue of subacute care is discussed in some detail in chapter six.

Medicare and Nursing Homes

One of the greatest expenses to the Medicare/Medicaid system is that of providing for the residents of nursing homes, typically – although there are many exceptions – elderly women with memory loss or dementia to varying degrees. Many are physically healthy for their age, but need help attending to hygiene and other personal needs, such as dressing and eating. The typical nursing home resident has managed to set aside around $20,000 for retirement, when the average annual cost of nursing home care is more than twice that much. This means that she (or he) can only pay for a stay of six months in a nursing home. The average stay is three years, and the resident becomes dependent on Medicaid and the modest income that social security provides. Residents' assets, in the form of material possessions, are taken into consideration in evaluating

Medicaid claims. These must not be worth more than $2000 to qualify for this form of state assistance.

Portrait of a Medicare Beneficiary

We must never forget that Medicare beneficiaries are not just statistics, or problems to be dealt with. Each recipient is a person. Somebody's father or mother, aunt or uncle, sister, brother or fellow citizen. I'd like to introduce you to Maria Sanchez, aged eighty-three, a Medicare Beneficiary, a mother of four and a former girl scout leader.

It is eight in the morning and Maria, who lives in Sunny Orchards nursing home in Florida, is being served breakfast by Anna-Mae, the nurses' aide assigned to the task. Maria suffers from Alzheimer's, and tends to be particularly confused in the mornings, although she regains much of her mental clarity when she wakes up properly. Between mouthfuls, she asks Anna Mae where her daughter Eileen is. Eileen died in a car accident over twenty-five years ago. Maria and Anna Mae have this conversation every morning.

Until she was seventy-five, Maria lived alone in the home that she had shared with her husband until his death. Maria and Carlos were typical, hard-working Americans – not overly concerned with wealth – and they were always able to make ends meet until they reached their seventies and began to experience health failure. In Carlos' case, this lead to his death of prostate cancer at the age of seventy-four. Maria had a series of non-serious but persistent health problems throughout her seventies. As she grew older, her conditions became worse, and the cost of medication soared. The few life savings that she and Carlos had worked so hard for were used up, and so were the social security payments. Medicare payments, although they covered a certain amount, were not enough to cover all of Maria's living expenses and healthcare needs, and as time passed, she began cutting corners – reducing grocery bills, telling the boy who always cut the lawn not to call round any more, and canceling her subscription to her favorite newspapers and magazines. Because she didn't mention her financial problems to them, some months passed before her children realized what was going on. Maria had lost twenty pounds in weight by the time she moved in with her son Dave and his wife Anna.

Things went smoothly for a while, but shortly after her eightieth birthday, Maria began to display symptoms of Alzheimer's disease, becoming increasingly disorientated and confused until one day she fell and broke her hip, necessitating hospitalization. She received good treatment there, but there was heavy pressure to discharge her, because Medicare would not pay for rehabilitation services in the hospital. There were two options. Maria could be sent home to her son's house, where she would receive home care services extending to one hour a day several days a week, or she could be discharged to a nursing home for therapy and continuing care.

The Sanchez family held a meeting and decided that the stress involved in caring for Maria was too much for Dave and Anna, and that it was time that their mother received professional care. The hospital had given them a list of nursing homes in the area, and the family set about going to visit them all. They didn't like what they saw. All of the facilities looked alike, with grim, tired staff, and depressed, ill at ease residents. The smallest home cared for only sixty people and looked more promising, but it was already full and there was a waiting list. What Maria was in need of was long-term care – somewhere to live until her time came to die. She would also be dependent on welfare payments to cover the cost of looking after her. Needless to say, the best nursing homes did not have a welfare vacancy – understandable, when one considers that the state reimburses them to the tune of $120 a day, while private pay homes charge $175. Dave, growing increasingly desperate to find somewhere safe and comfortable for his mother to live, offered to make up the difference, in order to allow Maria to move to one of the more pleasant facilities, but the director of the home told him that that would be impossible – in fact, according to the law, it's a crime! Another problem was the fact that Maria suffers from Alzheimer's disease. It's always harder to find a home for patients with this condition.

At last, a nursing home was found. It's not perfect, but it is reasonably close to Dave's house and it cares for only ninety patients. Maria is lucky to share a room with only one other woman. The room measures 12 feet by 12 feet, and the bathroom has one toilet and one sink. Each patient has a small bedside table and wall closet, but Maria has no room for her personal belongings, and no window to look out of.

The residents of Sunny Orchards nursing home are cared for by registered nurses, and by certified nurses' aides. The doctor drops by just once a month, because that is all that Medicare will pay for. When a resident needs to see a physician they are sent to the hospital emergency room. Maria spends almost all her time in bed, as she needs help to get up and to get back into bed. When she is not lying down, she is usually in a wheelchair. Although her broken hip mended, her therapy did not make her mobile enough to walk long distances. Dave feels that the nursing home is responsible in not providing enough physical therapy for his mother. When she was first transferred, a physical therapist conducted an evaluation and started daily therapy. This lasted for a month, or something less than 15 hours in total, at which stage the therapist said that she wouldn't benefit from any more.

Now, several months later, Maria has settled into a regular routine. The day begins at 7 when the morning shift of nurses starts work. Breakfast is served in bed every morning by a nurse who also has to feed another seven residents, each of whom has about 15 minutes to finish the meal. When Carlos was alive, they would eat together, talking about the events of the day. Now, even though she is confused, Maria wonders why she can't eat in the dining room, where she would be able to sit with other residents and chat a little. The nurses are always so busy that they have very little time to spend talking to her, barely managing to finish the basics of helping her to sit up, attend to her toilet, and get settled into her wheelchair. Last year, Maria grew very fond of LaBelle, a young nurses' aide, but LaBelle developed repetitive strain injury and had to seek employment elsewhere.

Most mornings, Maria sits either in her room or in a hallway or day room until lunch is ready. On some days the activity director organizes something for the residents to do, but Maria is not able to cope with taking part. Lunch is served in shifts, as the dining room isn't big enough for all the patients. Sometimes Maria eats at noon, and sometimes half an hour later.

Maria's family is concerned. Although most of the caregivers seem to be dedicated professionals, there have been some worrying incidents in the nursing home. Last week, an elderly man broke his wrist as he struggled to release himself from the restraints that held him to his wheelchair. A month before, Maria was found to be suffering from a pressure sore. Dave and Sarah held a meeting with the nursing home director, who apologized, but told them that he just could not afford to hire more staff to care for his patients.

The service provided in Sunny Orchards nursing home is not good enough. But although her family has searched far and wide for a better placement for Maria, there doesn't seem to be anywhere else. Stress levels among all the children are growing, and it is hard to know who to be angry with. The nurses' aides who didn't turn Maria often enough because they were short of help and too busy to stop and help her change position? Should they blame themselves, for committing her to a nursing home? The nursing home director who is only just managing to break even at the end of the financial year? The last time that Dave saw his mother, she had one of her few lucid moments.

"I want to die," she told him, "living here is not a life."

CHAPTER TWO:
MY INTRODUCTION TO THE
NURSING HOME INDUSTRY

I started working in the healthcare system when Medicare and Medicaid were new, and throughout my professional life, I've watched the ebbs and flows in healthcare in the United States. From nursing and administration to owning my own establishment, my professional journey throughout the last three decades is also, to a large extent, the story of the United States healthcare system in the latter part of the twentieth century and the opening years of the new millennium. I offer an insight to my own experiences to you so that you will how healthcare works, from the point of view of those intimately involved in its daily administration.

Early Days

I was born in Chico, California on June 5th, 1943, to Francis Hope Burr and Guy Rice Seaton – for whom I was named – but I was raised, along with my two brothers and my sister, in Hot Springs, Arkansas. My grandfather, Guy Ralph Seaton, was sexton of Greenwood Cemetery there, and Dad worked with him in maintenance, eventually replacing his father as sexton when he passed away following a heart attack. My childhood was unexceptional – its details would be familiar to any lower middle-class American family. I achieved average grades in school, and enjoyed all the activities then available to a young boy – baseball, basketball, boxing and just hanging out. On graduating from high school in 1961, I joined the army for a term of three years, and after basic training was assigned to the 3rd armor cavalry unit in Kaiserlautern, Germany. During this period, I rose to the rank of specialist fourth class, company clerk.

On returning to the United States I started looking for work and thinking about attending the University of Arkansas, but without money for tuition, it seemed wise to take up my grandmother's offer to go and live with her in California, where there were opportunities to develop. There, I applied and was accepted for a state employee position as a psychiatric technician.

At that time – in 1965 – my grandmother was employed at Modesto State Hospital. She worked the night-shift, caring for those patients with long-term conditions. In those days, the mentally ill and disabled had few rights. They were invariably taken from the community and locked in state hospitals, and caring for them was stressful, arduous work. My training took place at Stockton State Hospital. Tired of the daily commute from my grandmother's home, I moved to Stockton for the duration of my education.

At this time, the professionals who cared for the mentally ill in California were know as "psychiatric technicians". They were trained in the administration of medication, nursing treatment procedures and psychiatric nursing. This was my first exposure to the American healthcare system, and to the needs of people in acute, chronic crisis. Those cared for in the system were diverse, including those with chronic brain disease, and both psychotherapy and drugs were used to control the patients whose behavior had spiraled out of control. In this context, I learned the importance of interpersonal relationships in keeping both the mind and the body well. After one year of initial training, I was assigned to Stockton State Hospital, where I divided my time between working and attending courses. Another year later, I was promoted to the position of shift supervisor, and offered a job at the Sonoma State Hospital in California. Working at night, I attended the San Rosa Junior College during the day, and was accepted, after two further years of study, to the Sonoma State University, where I earned a degree in management. During my senior year, I received an internship in Hospital Administration, and after graduation I passed the necessary examination to hold a nursing home administrator license.

The late 1960s and early 1970s were formative years in my career, and they were also important years in the evolution of the American healthcare system. Profound changes were occurring in the field at this time. Medicare was introduced, creating new opportunities for the elderly to be cared for in skilled nursing facilities, extended care facilities or nursing homes and to receive the rehabilitation necessary to allow them to return home. At the same time, a quiet revolution was under way in the area of mental healthcare. Patients were being moved from psychiatric facilities to local community mental health programs and long-term psychiatric

My Introduction to the Nursing Home Industry

nursing homes, because Medicare and Medicaid began to pay for these services. Prior to these sweeping reforms, all nursing homes were independently owned, and cared for private patients. They were licensed, but state regulations were weak and unspecific. Medicare regulations were passed, which reflected basic operational requirements. For example, each home had to incorporate a governing body, and provide a nursing service, a physical plant, infection control, and a utilization review.

As psychiatric patients moved from state hospitals to community based programs, the opportunity arose for me to take a position as supervisor at the Sonoma State Hospital for the mentally retarded. At this time, the use of the term "developmentally disabled" became common to describe such people and, for the first time, the federal government, under the Medicare system, began to help to pay for the care and treatment of them in the context of a nursing home.

When federal government began to pay for extended care benefits of 100 days of post-hospital care, the response across the nation was the mushrooming of skilled nursing facilities, nursing homes and convalescent hospitals. Nursing management companies were created almost overnight. New facilities were being built, and privately held nursing homes were acquired. Suddenly, nursing homes were big business!

While this expansion took place, I was attending Sonoma State University as a Management major. Sonoma didn't offer the usual courses in business administration as it was then taught, but a new and innovative approach to business – management. As well as offering accountancy and finance courses, the school placed a strong emphasis on humanistic management. With a background in healthcare, I found this fascinating, and took course work that taught me about the social, interpersonal approach to managing a workforce. This new approach to business resembled the new approach to psychiatry in one very important way: for the first time, the humanity of individuals was being recognized.

As I worked in the state hospital system, which was administered along the lines of a hospital organization, I decided to try to obtain training in hospital administration. Course work in this area was not offered, but I was also following a course of studies in political science, and this department offered an internment class for two semesters. On meeting with the hospital administrator at Sonoma State Hospital, I proposed myself as an intern, if he would agree to be my preceptor.

This was my first experience of witnessing how a hospital worked from the very highest levels of authority. During my internship, I learned about all of the hospital's departments – maintenance, infection control, general services. I worked as supervisor of general services for a brief period, and also conducted studies and worked with the administrator on various projects, one of which was preparing the hospital for certification under the Medicare program for reimbursement. During this time, I became versed in the regulations and requirements of a skilled nursing facility, and interested in moving into the area of administration on graduation, or possibly attending graduate school to study hospital administration.

When I graduated in 1973, I applied for a position as the administrator of a 99-bed nursing home called Pacific Convalescent hospital in Oakland, California, one of a small chain of six facilities located in the Bay Area. Although my only experience at this point was my internship and some exposure to supervising three other employees, I was hired. Nursing home administrators were rare, as the state had passed a licensing law requiring all such people to pass an examination and to be licensed in the state of California. I had passed this examination in my senior year. Many nursing home owners had never taken the necessary examination, and were obliged to hire administrators. At this point in time, administrators were not very highly paid – I received around $800 a month, less than I had earned as an employee of the state hospital system. Nonetheless, fresh from school with new ideas of management and motivating the work force, I embarked on my new career with enthusiasm, as did my counterparts all over the country. There was still no specific education program for training nursing home administrators. Most had acquired on the job experience, or had worked as interns for 1,000 hours before taking the necessary examination.

Looking back after more than three decades in the industry, I can see that I was largely unprepared for the challenges that I faced as an administrator. First of all, the nursing home had no director of nurses, and the nursing department was short-staffed – conditions that still prevail at many nursing homes today. And that wasn't all. Somehow, the accounting department was unable to send the necessary documentation to Medicare and Medicaid when and as necessary.

I will never forget the smell of the facility when I started working there. Although it was less than six years old, the entire building had a lingering, foul odor. I now know that this smell is common throughout the nursing home industry. It is caused by decaying bacteria pooled in urine that has not been cleaned properly from beds, rails, floors, mattresses and equipment. Many homes try to mask the smell with perfumed air sprays, but this measure just makes it all the more offensive. I made my first goal the elimination of the smell from the home.

Despite the odor, I was pleased to find the managers and employees friendly, helpful and apparently dedicated and hardworking. This was some consolation, as I was anxious about my new role. I was to be responsible for ninety-nine elderly patients in a home that was understaffed and experiencing financial difficulty. I was also relieved by the professionalism of my supervisor, Mrs. Laura Harr, a dedicated registered nurse who would not tolerate any lowering of the quality of care. She was overworked and supervised six skilled nursing facility administrators, but she understood the field from every possible angle and provided support and encouragement. She didn't know me, and took a risk in working with me. I resolved not to disappoint her.

Believing in a participatory management, one of the first things I did was to gather the supervisors around and discuss my general approach. Daily meetings with supervisors were instigated, at which they could discuss their problems, inform others and propose solutions to difficult issues. Instead of seeking a director of nurses from outside the organization, I offered the position to a registered nurse who was the day shift charge nurse. She was apprehensive, but welcomed the opportunity to learn and expand her talents. I think that the fact that we were both new and learning as we went along helped us to improve the quality of care.

But first things first! Together with the housekeeping supervisor, I worked out a cleaning schedule to ensure that all equipment and bedding would be washed every day. We had to count on the cooperation of the nursing department, as patients had to be out of bed before sheets were changed, and bedding cleaned. Despite the extra expense and increased workload in the laundry, I decided that bed linen should be cleaned on a daily basis. The unpleasant odor was gone in a matter of weeks.

Although nursing homes were not required to seek accreditation from the Joint Commission of Accreditation of hospitals (now the Joint Commission of Accreditation of Healthcare Organizations) [7], I proposed taking this step, although the supervisors were afraid that we wouldn't be up to the challenge. I assured them that if we really tried, we could be, and they reluctantly applied themselves to the task of meeting the challenging standards. Six months later, we applied for accreditation, received an onsite inspection, and made the grade! Although we still had some distance to travel in creating the type of nursing facility we aspired to run, all of us were proud that we had worked as a team, improved the quality of our care, and achieved recognition from a national organization. Not long afterwards, we passed the annual state and Medicare survey without any deficiencies. We were off to a good start.

---

[7] In 1951, the American College of Physicians, the American Hospital Association, the American Medical Association and the Canadian Medical Association joined the American College of Surgeons in formally launching the Joint Commission of Accreditation of Hospitals. This organization has played an important role in advancing patient safety and the quality of healthcare both in North America and around the world, being consistently on the cutting edge of developing new methods both for evaluating the performance of healthcare organizations and for helping these in improving the quality of care they provide.

CHAPTER THREE:
THE HEALTHCARE ARMY

It takes a lot of people to run a nursing home – members of the public are often surprised by just how many different types of heath-care professional there are! From the basic care given by nurses' aides, to the highly specialized service of people such as physiotherapists and dieticians, an army – even if it is an under-staffed one – of personnel provides for the needs of America's elders.

Not every nursing facility has a full complement of healthcare workers, but every well run institution is organized into the following departments or services; administration, nursing, staff development or in-service director, dietary or food services, activities, medical records, housekeeping and laundry, maintenance, fire safety, occupational health, material management, social services, physical therapy, speech therapy, occupational therapy, pharmacy services and consultant services. Each department is headed by a supervisor, and each distinct service is usually provided by only one or two individuals, according to the size of the home. Smaller homes may have personnel who fill more than one role at the same time. Many nursing homes do not have an in-house medical staff, but all must have a physician who acts as the medical director. Each department or service has policies and procedures that provide detailed instructions as to how services should be carried out. These are the same in all nursing homes, as they are based on the federal rules and regulations governing such institutions. Many nursing homes provide the minimum quality of care possible while implementing these rules for a combination of reasons. In the case of homes owned by large corporations, their chief motivation is to keep the investors happy – not the residents.

The staff enumerated in this chapter is hired by a majority of institutions in order to comply with federal, state and local standards and with all the guidelines and regulations that govern nursing homes. Compliance with federal and state regulations is the first priority – not the health and well being of the residents. Thus, the services offered by employees are designed to prevent any infringement of the rules, leaving little room for flexibility and the tailoring of healthcare to individual needs. Nursing home employees, from the most highly qualified and specialized to those providing the most basic, hands-on care, soon learn that Medicare and licensing inspectors are, quite simply, referred to as "the state". They learn that their job is to satisfy the health inspectors and not help the residents to make the most of their lives. Many spend more time ensuring that paperwork is in order than providing basic healthcare services to those whom they have been employed to look after.

Please don't misunderstand me – I am not suggesting that nursing homes should be unregulated. But we must understand that human beings do not operate according to fixed rules. Everybody is different, and our uniqueness does not fade with the passage of time. Residents should, when necessary, be able to avail of services and care not covered by the all-powerful regulations, and employees should be assured that, in all cases, the needs of the resident are more important than compliance with the rules. That said, let's proceed and examine the role of the many different types of nursing home employee. Bear in mind that, in many cases, one person fulfills two or more of the categories I discuss below.

Administration

Nursing homes have complex, multi-faceted roles in society today. Nursing and other medical staff have more than enough to do taking care of the patients. But who co-ordinates and organizes everything? Every business needs an administrative body, and nursing homes are no exception to this rule.

Each nursing home operates under the auspices of a governing body, which bears the legal responsibility for establishing and implementing policies regarding management. It is this body that appoints a state-licensed administrator who will take care of the facility's management issues. The administration as a whole is responsible for the presence of a disaster and emergency preparedness plan to cover all potential problems, from fire to missing residents. It must ensure that employees are trained in emergency procedures and conduct unannounced staff drills. An important aspect of administration is the presence of a quality assessment and assurance committee consisting of the director of nursing services, a physician and at least three other members of staff. The committee is responsible for identifying ways of improving the quality of care in the nursing home. Every nursing facility depends on its administrative staff for the smooth day-to-day running of the home. The role of the nursing home administrator is just what the title implies. He or she – invariably a person licensed by the state to work as a nursing home administrator – directs the day-to-day functioning of the home to ensure that it complies with federal, state and local standards. Administrators are required to obtain a license in accordance with state and local law in order to operate a nursing home. The principal duties and responsibilities of the administrator fall within the following categories: committee functions, personnel functions, staff development, safety and sanitation equipment, supply, budget and planning functions and finally, residents' rights. As well as ensuring that all of these regulations are met, administrators must not discriminate on the basis of age, race, color or national origin. They co-ordinate the workers, decide and implement policy and make important decisions about personnel, finance, facility operations, and admissions, being responsible for employing qualified personnel to provide all of the services required, including laboratory services, radiology and x-ray services. The administrator serves on various committees of the institution including hospital, quality control and assessment, utilization review and pharmaceutical and budget committees. Committees make recommendations as to the implementation of policy, and these are reviewed and discussed with management. Decisions must comply with federal, state and local standards and with the guidelines and regulations that govern the institution, and they are implemented so long as they are consistent with the goals and budget of the organization.

Nursing home administrators were formerly drawn from the ranks of those with nursing or other medical qualifications. Increasingly, they have business backgrounds – vital for running a nursing home in today's economic environment. While every facility has a general administrator, larger homes may have specialized administrators in charge of the various departments. In smaller facilities, top administrators handle many of the details of daily operation. All administrators must pass a state and national licensing examination and hold a valid license in order to work. To qualify for the examination, candidates must have earned a degree from an accredited college or university, and have completed 1,000 hours of training in a nursing home beneath of the supervision of a preceptor who is also an administrator.

As the healthcare system develops and becomes ever more complex, administrators will have to become more adept at managing integrated healthcare delivery systems, new technological innovations and increased demands for efficiency. Many do not have the academic background and support to manage the changes that the introduction of subacute care will bring. Only some administrators hold advanced degrees in health services administration, long-term care administration, health sciences, public health, public administration or business services administration. Needless to say, although hands-on experience is an important aspect of becoming a competent administrator, one should also be grounded in academic theories of long-term care and management. One of my personal disappointments is that, even now, neither the industry nor the government requires a uniform course of study in a higher academic education program in order to become a nursing home administrator, despite the stringent requirements demanded of other types of healthcare professional. Currently, nursing home administrators are from a range of academic backgrounds including social science, the liberal arts, accounting, business, political science, public administration and more. If nursing homes are to offer a full service and become more than simply compliant with federal and state rules, administrators *must* have backgrounds in business and management. These skills are vital to the successful functioning of a nursing home in today's economic environment. America's failure to provide adequate training for nursing home administrators reflects the low esteem with which nursing professionals are generally viewed.

While every facility has an administrator who is in charge of the entire nursing home, each department is headed by a supervisor, from the business office, kitchen, housekeeping and laundry to nursing services, medical records, maintenance, social services and activities. Directors of nursing must be trained professionals, but other supervisory positions have no minimum education requirement. One should be at least a high school graduate, with additional training or experience of at least a year or two in the field. The reason for the low educational standards is simple: money. College graduates expect to earn more, and to enter a career where they can advance both financially and professionally. Healthcare does not offer these possibilities, and many of these positions become dead end jobs, with little opportunity to gain salary increases in line with inflation.

Larger facilities can have several assistant administrators to help the top administrator handle the day-to-day operation of the home or institution. They may be assigned specialist duties in coordinating the efforts of nurses, therapists, clerks, accountants, etc. Many are top administrators in the making, and this is where they learn their craft. Typical duties include financial management and helping with the development of job descriptions, assisting the director of nurses and other supervisors in carrying out their duties, attending committee meetings, carrying out committee functions and helping with the recruitment of personnel and other personnel issues.

The role of the patient care advocate in the nursing home is to ensure that residents are receiving the care they need, and to mediate between residents and their families and the caregivers. Among their duties are confirming appointments and informing patients of information that they may need, clarifying and reviewing immunization reports, working closely with health providers, making appointments and investigating queries and complaints

Patient care advocates are arranged privately by each institution, and unless the government states explicitly that such a position must be filled, most nursing homes will not ensure that it is. Despite the benefits that a patient care advocate brings to a nursing organization, many managers see the role as an unnecessary expense and one must always try to find out whether the position has been filled before arranging to have a resident admitted. Managers tend to feel that the nurse and the administration are themselves the advocates of the patients, with each employee trained in protecting patients' rights. The case study below illustrates clearly how, even with the best will in the world, the regular nursing staff and administration do not necessarily always provide the most complete service possible.

Case Study

Appian nursing home is one of the few such institutions in its area to employ its own patient care advocate. It's not cheap, hiring an extra employee to watch over patients' rights, but earlier this year the wisdom behind the move was made abundantly clear. Evelyn O'Brien, a resident in her late 70s, had a tendency towards hypochondria, claiming that she was ill in order to obtain the attention from the nursing staff that she craved. Nurses and physicians alike had grown used to taking her complaints with a pinch of salt. Although not strong, her general physical health had always been quite stable, and too many times she had been admitted to hospital for suspected heart problems only to be released with a diagnosis of indigestion. Hypochondriac patients are often the most difficult of all to deal with – it's so hard to tell when they are really ill and when it's largely in their minds. They usually can't even tell themselves.

When Evelyn began to complain of discomfort in her back and chest in February, the home physician took a quick look at her, and decided that she was probably suffering from the same old complaint – slight indigestion exacerbated by hypochondria. She diagnosed some indigestion tablets, and moved on to examine more profoundly ill patients. Evelyn's family, always realistic about their mother's tendency to exaggerate, were nonetheless sure that this time was different. They spoke to the charge nurse and the director of nurses, both of whom said they'd look into the matter, but reminded them that Evelyn had just been seen by the facility's physician. The director of nurses suggested that they discuss their problem with the home's patient care advocate.

Giovanni Nuttall listened carefully to everything that they had to say. He gently reminded the O'Briens of Evelyn's tendency to exaggerate, but promised to ensure that she would be reexamined with more attention to detail. The first thing he did was to contact the director of nurses and charge nurse to discuss the O'Brien's concerns. In response, the director of nurses arranged, through the attending physician, for Evelyn to be seen by another doctor. The consultant discovered that Evelyn was presenting with the early symptoms of angina, a heart complaint that affects many elderly people, but which can be controlled quite well in most cases with the right medication. Evelyn is now taking a course of medicines to help her cope with the new condition and has changed her meal schedule from three large meals a day to a number of snacks. The angina seems to have stabilized, and she is able to take part in the activities she always enjoyed. This case is an excellent example of the value of the patient care advocate in the nursing home – by intervening, Giovanni was able to prompt the physician to take another look at Evelyn and reassure the family that their mother's health was, indeed, being carefully monitored. It is quite likely that this intervention prevented Evelyn from developing a more serious, more distressing and more costly complaint.

Every business needs reliable secretarial staff, and nursing homes are no exception to this rule. Secretaries fulfill the usual important tasks of typing, filing, handling correspondence and calendars, checking appointments and taking care of all the details that go into the smooth functioning of an office. Secretaries may be assigned specialist duties such as processing admissions and coordinating the efforts of nurses, therapists, clerks, accountants, etc.

Accountants and bookkeepers form an essential part of every nursing home's administration team. Depending on their size, homes employ a business office manager and from one to four accounting clerks or bookkeepers. Among their duties is taking care of the payroll and bill for services to Medicare, Medicaid, Insurance Companies, HMOs and private patients. Accountants are the most well informed on the financial operation of the nursing home, and must be able to answer any queries about Medicare and Medicaid payment or the coinsurance requirements of any given resident.

Nursing Department

Nurses and their assistants form the bulk of a nursing home's staff, and they represent the heart of any nursing home, with the largest number of employees of any department, including certified nurses' assistants, registered nurses, licensed vocational nurses and ward clerks. The director of nurses must be a registered nurse possessed of organizational skills and developed managerial qualities.

The nursing service of a nursing home is required by federal regulations to "... have sufficient staff to provide nursing and related services to attain or maintain the highest practicable physical, mental and psychosocial well being of each resident, as determined by resident assessments and individual plans of care." Sufficient nursing staff – what does this mean? The federal regulations are unclear. Instead of giving specific guidelines as to appropriate staff/resident ratios, they state that "the facility must provide services in sufficient numbers to each of the following types of personnel on a 24 hour basis to provide nursing care to all residents in accordance with resident care plans." The only requisites are that one licensed nurse should serve as a charge nurse on each tour of duty. This person may be a licensed vocational or practical nurse, or a registered nurse. Nursing homes are supposed to use the services of a registered nurse for at least eight consecutive hours a day, seven days a week, although this regulation can be waived under certain conditions, including notifying residents and their immediate families of the waiver. In the absence of clear staffing regulations, nursing home owners, be they private or corporate, "solve" their staffing issues by employing as many as can be paid for by the institution's revenue, and *no more*. Payments for services are not based upon assessment of residents and individual plans of care, and the nursing departments of healthcare facilities are routinely understaffed.

The director of nurses must be a registered nurse licensed by the state with at least one year's experience as a charge nurse. Many homes also require directors to hold a nursing degree from an accredited college or university, but such a qualification is not mandatory. Nurses must have graduated from a nursing program and passed a national licensing examination, and in some states they are required to take ongoing courses in order to ensure the renewal of their license. Experience in the field is the primary qualification, however, as is willingness to be responsible for the care of nursing home residents. The director of nurses is in charge of the entire staff of nurses' assistants, registered nurses, licensed vocational nurses and ward clerks. The director must ensure that each resident receives the necessary care, and take responsibility for staffing the facility within the staff ratio and budget allowed by the corporation or the private owner. The current federal, state and local standards, guidelines and regulations must always be borne in mind. As well as taking care of administrative duties, the director of nurses is assigned to care plan and assessment functions. He or she must also oversee staff development, infection control, utilization review, safety issues and the ordering of nursing supplies and equipment, while ensuring that all the services required by residents are obtained, including social services, activities and physicians' visits. Most of his or her time is spent recruiting and staffing the facility, and in dealing with requests from nurses and other staff for time off. The director of nurses is also a member of all the home's committees and must attend meetings and contribute to decision taking. He or she relies heavily upon charge nurses and other nursing staff to ensure that infection control, patients' rights, utilization control and admission and discharge plans are developed and up-to-date. The director should be able to guarantee that a basic level of care is provided by nurses' assistants, that medications are given to patients correctly and in a timely manner, that the residents' state of health is reported to the physician, and that their daily care is documented as a medical record. The director of nurses may have an assistant and other key personnel to take care of the details of all of the above tasks, but he or she is ultimately responsible. The most difficult tasks facing any director are recruiting staff, preventing existing staff from leaving, and ensuring that nurses show up for work. The nursing home relies heavily on this key employee, as the type and quality of care that a nursing facility can offer are directly related to the director of nurses' ability to manage and direct, including arranging for the ongoing education of the nursing home staff. The director of nurses works in close collaboration with the business office and all other support departments, including housekeeping, food service, maintenance, and direct treatment staff comprising physical therapists, occupational therapists, speech therapists, consultant physicians and psychologists. Charge nurses and other support staff must be trusted to monitor infection control, patient rights and utilization control and to ensure that admission and discharge plans are developed and kept up-to-date, but all answer to the director of nurses, whose responsibility it is to ensure that everyone is cared for, and that everything is documented.

As in the case of nursing home administrators, the director of nurses is always preoccupied with the current federal, state and local standard guidelines and regulations governing nursing homes. Directors of nurses face an almost impossible task on a daily basis. It's not surprising that they are sometimes referred to as "super nurses".

Case Study: Portrait of a Director of Nurses

Sinead Fulcher is the director of nurses in Liberty Hall nursing home, an establishment that was recently purchased by a large nursing home chain. Sinead graduated from one of her state's best nursing schools and quickly rose through the ranks to become a director of nurses at only 28 years of age. Although she is the mother of 18 month old twins, she is never distracted from the many duties that her job brings – healthcare provider, diplomat, paperwork expert and more. She takes us through an average day's work.

"After dropping my sons off at their daycare center, I arrive at work at 9 a.m. and get busy straight away, reviewing the reports left by the night staff. If any of the residents has had a change in condition during the night, it may be necessary to review their medications and for that, we need to make sure they see a physician, either here or in the nearby hospital.

By the time I arrive at work, the morning shift of nurses' aides and charge nurses has already been in for an hour or more, serving breakfasts and attending to residents' needs. I feel sorry for the nurses' aides, because they are paid at a very low rate – and sorry for myself, because I have to keep filling their positions as they become vacant. We have a huge turnover in nurses' aides and more than once I've been forced to hire someone I didn't feel was right for the job out of sheer desperation!

Monday is always a big day for meetings – at various times throughout the day, the different committees meet to discuss infection control, the development of care plans and all the other issues that the top level of nursing home staff has to cover. Sometimes, meetings just last for minutes but on other days they can go on for hours, as we thrash through the practical and bureaucratic issues involved in keeping everything running smoothly. On those occasions, I get behind at keeping paperwork up-to-date, and have to work extra hard on Tuesday and Wednesday to catch up.

Most days, I spend some time talking to residents' families. I like to give them as much time as I can, especially those who have recently left their mother or father with us. Families always have understandable concerns about how we'll look after their parent or relative and I try to answer all the questions and settle any problems that arise. Some people, burdened with feelings of guilt and anxiety, lash out about the slightest thing and I can get frustrated at times with families who demand everything of the nursing staff without giving anything back in terms of background information or support. Part of my job is to keep a pleasant expression on my face at all times, and answer every question and complaint with dignity. Fortunately, I'm blessed with an excellent assistant, Gladys Mannix, who really is my right hand! She's been a nurse for over 30 years, and brings a wonderful air of serenity to the job. I usually get annoyed when people describe nurses as having a "vocation" – often a sly way of diminishing their professionalism – but in her case, the term does apply.

By 5 p.m., I'm more than ready to leave, but I often end up working one or more hours overtime, as I struggle to leave everything in order for the next day. Fortunately, my husband Jim is a teacher – he finishes work at 4 so he can pick the kids from daycare, bring them home and see that they have something to eat. Despite all the drawbacks to my job, I'm glad that I became a nurse, and that I worked hard to become a director. Several of the homes owned by the chain that recently bought Liberty Hall have had enormous problems, with cases of neglect brought to light. We're facing our own difficulties here, with budget cuts promised for the near future, but at least I know that, if any resident has good reason to complain, it won't be because I wasn't doing my best to make their final years pleasant ones

Am I glad I went into nursing? Well yes, I am. But, I have to say, unless things improve a *lot* in the future, I'm not going to recommend it as a career to my two little boys when they grow up! I'd rather they were teachers like Jim. He says his job is difficult and stressful, but he'd soon stop complaining if he had to take over from me for a week or two.

Homes with at least 100 beds hire an assistant director of nurses – it's unusual for a home with fewer residents to do so, especially those smaller homes with under 60 beds. This staff member works as the nursing director's second hand, helping him or her with the duties of running the home. The assistant may be assigned the functions of infection control, staff development and the training of nurses' assistants, as well as the direct supervision of nurses' assistants, and licensed medication and treatment nurses.

Nursing homes with less than 60 beds usually have only one registered nurse on duty on any given day – generally speaking, the director of nurses. When the director of nurses is also the only registered nurse on hand, he or she must combine the clinical duties of the position with the administrative and managerial ones.

Registered nurses' clinical duties are to identify disease and other health problems so far as possible, promote health and help patients by observing, assessing and recording symptoms, reactions and progress. They administer medications, work with patients who are convalescing or undergoing rehabilitation and cooperate closely with residents' physicians. They also develop treatment plans, supervise licensed practical nurses and nurses' aides and operate skilled procedures such as intravenous feeding and catheterization. Medium sized nursing homes (from 60 to 100 beds) are obliged to hire registered or licensed nurses to carry out clinical duties including medication, assessment and charting. Of all the nursing home employees working in the institution on a full-time basis, the registered nurses are the ones with the most advanced level of medical training. Only those homes with at least 100 beds ensure that there is a registered nurse on duty at all times.

A charge nurse is assigned to each nursing shift. In smaller homes, with less than 100 beds, charge nurses are often licensed vocational or practical nurses, while the are more frequently registered nurses in the larger homes. A charge nurse is the director of nurses' second hand, helping him or her with the duties of running the home. This nursing home employee is the most underrated of all, usually being in charge of an entire nursing home, or an entire station if the home has more than one. She (it may be a man, but is more frequently a woman) must supervise the nurses' aides and ensure that they are performing all their duties satisfactorily. She must also answer the phone, speak with family members, take orders from her superiors and report any change in residents' conditions to the attending physician and family members. She is responsible for coordinating all of the activities of the nursing home or station, and dealing with any problems that arise. Often she must also administer mediation and treatments, and more than once in a while she has to take over the duties of other nurses who take shifts off – a common scenario is for evening shift nurses to receive a call from the night shift nurse to say that she's not coming to work. When this happens, the charge nurse has to find a replacement or be prepared to cover the shift by working overtime. Charge nurses have to handle the delicate task of managing problems with employees and complaints from both residents and family members. A charge nurse is obliged to visit every resident in her daily watch in order to conduct an assessment – although if one resident needs special attention the others may not receive all the care they need. Emergencies always have to be dealt with first. As well as providing hands-on administration and nursing care, the charge nurse has to be careful to keep up-to-date with paperwork. She has to ensure that all the nurses' aides have been charted, and that medication and treatments have been recorded and accounted for. Filling in the forms can take a long time, and divert her from providing real patient care but to avoid a bureaucratic nightmare later on, it's very important. Officially speaking, whatever hasn't been documented hasn't been done! She's often so busy, that she doesn't find time to have lunch, and just grabs a coffee and a sandwich at the nurses' station.

Case Study: Portrait of a Charge Nurse

Lisa Jovencito is originally from the Philippines, although she has been living and working in the United States for more than fifteen years. As a young girl, she had hoped to go into psychiatry, but she was from a large family and there just wasn't enough money to put her through college. When a friend suggested that she might enjoy nursing, she wasn't sure, but after a few years she realized that she enjoyed making a difference to the lives of the sick and vulnerable. Nurses can earn much more in the United States than in the Philippines, so Lisa moved, but she regularly sends money home to help with the education of her young nieces and nephews.

> I'm a registered nurse, and so I hope that some day I'll be a director of nurses, but I haven't got that far yet! My official title in the home where I work is "Charge Nurse and Night Supervisor". I'm in charge of ninety-nine patients, and provide nursing care for them during the night. One of the tasks that takes up most of my time is supervising the nurses' aides. I have some excellent workers on my ward, but there are always a few who are inclined not to bathe residents, or to rush through meals. There's never enough time to get through these duties as calmly as I'd like, and I often have to roll up my sleeves and help the nurses' aides get everyone clean and dressed. Of course, the aides can't administer medications and monitor the intravenous tubes, so I do all of that for myself. I always try to talk to the patients as much as possible, especially those who either have no families, or who rarely receive visits. I think being so far from home gives me an insight into how overwhelming loneliness can be. As the only registered nurse who works the night shift, I have to assess patients during the night and decide when and if a doctor should be called. When someone passes away, it's my responsibility to contact the coroner. Nursing can be rewarding, especially when patients, their families and physicians take the time to remember me and thank me for my efforts, but there are times when I just feel like I'm invisible. Do have any regrets? I wish that there had been enough money when I left high school to become a physician or psychiatrist, but at least one of my nieces is planning to go into medicine, so I know that the investment I'm making in her education is worthwhile.

Licensed practical or vocational nurses receive limited training – usually one year of clinical training with classroom work – and hold a license from the state. In many homes, these are the people who give medication and basic treatment to residents, as well as monitoring their health status. Many nursing homes with a hundred beds or less hire licensed practical nurses or vocational and charge nurses instead of registered nurses in order to keep costs down, as Medicare regulations only require facilities with more than a hundred beds to have a registered nurse on duty on each shift rather than just the day shift. Very small homes, with less than sixty beds, can have a charge nurse as director of nurses. Without licensed practical nurses, most institutions would have no employees with the skills necessary to assess and monitor residents on duty in the evenings and nights. Most nursing homes require licensed practical nurses to administer medication and treatments and effectively perform the duties of the charge nurse although, because their training is less advanced, they cannot be paid at the same rate. The workload of the licensed practical nurse is very heavy, as many residents become ill during the evening and night shifts and do not receive proper treatment until the following morning – not because the nurses don't care, but because they are occupied in handing out medicine, giving treatments, supervising nurses' aides and coping with staff shortages, charting and unforeseen incidents.

Certified nurses' aides are key workers who have undergone basic nursing training and provide much of the hands-on care, washing residents and helping them visit the toilet, eat their meals, dress and get in and out of bed and dealing with the daily chores of cleaning up feces, urine and vomit. These are the healthcare workers who have the most contact with nursing home residents, and the well being of these old people depends largely on the quality of the relationship they develop with the nurses' aides who care for them. They care for confused residents with behavioral problems who may become violent, they lift overweight residents in and out of bed ... their work is never-ending. Nurses' assistants or aides are the healthcare workers with the least formal training, and they receive the lowest pay. At the time of writing, a majority belongs to one ethnic minority or another, including Asians, Hispanics, Haitians and African-Americans. The problems that face this particular group of workers are immense, and are discussed in some detail under various headings throughout the book.

Nursing homes are required to incorporate a restorative program into their nursing services, intended to ensure that residents maintain and maximize their abilities, to increase resident independence and to minimize the problems caused by their disabilities. Many nursing homes put these duties in the hands of the certified nurses' aides, but progressive homes employ a licensed vocational or registered nurse to act as a restorative care nurse, and oversee the implementation of restorative care plans by the nurses' aides. Other homes may develop a restorative care program with the help of the physical therapist, occupational therapist or speech therapist in devising treatment programs which can be continued after the resident has stopped receiving therapy services. Restorative care functions include providing training in walking, in performing activities, and in a range of exercises designed to improve mobility and strength and other functions involving mounting or descending steps, and using supportive equipment.

Continuous education for nursing staff and other nursing home employees is important in maintaining the quality of the service providing, and the staff development director or instructor oversees precisely that. There are no overall standards as to how much ongoing education should be received by staff and, consequently, a majority of nursing homes does not provide more than token in-service education. Usually, a full-time staff member such as a registered or licensed vocational nurse with duties such as infection control or quality assessment is also required to oversee education. This person is responsible for planning and conducting education programs focusing on nursing policies and procedure, infection control and general care and treatment. New employees, especially, must undergo an orientation program before they begin work, comprising familiarity with the facilities, fire safety, policies and procedures, residents' rights and knowledge of the precautions that must be taken with respect to exposure to blood or other body fluids.

Food Service

Running a home involves more than medical care – residents have to be provided with meals three times a day, so a full kitchen staff is necessary. But that's not all. Meals have to be designed for elderly digestive systems, and for people who have specific nutritional needs. Menus, however, must be prepared within the cost range allotted by the home – costs have to be contained. Meals are nutritious, but are prepared with inexpensive meat, fish and chicken. Let's examine all the workers behind every nursing home meal.

Nursing home meals are designed around a menu developed by registered dieticians. Homes usually hire dieticians on a consultant basis, although they may also be employed either full- or part-time. Menus are usually ordered in advance, often on a quarterly basis, while individual patient's diets are ordered by the physician attending the residents. Dieticians plan nutrition programs, and supervise the preparation and serving of meals. By promoting healthy eating habits, and tailoring menus to individual residents' needs, they help to prevent and treat illness. As well as working with the food preparation staff, they consult with physicians, nurses and other medical staff to coordinate medical and dietary requirements. Planned meals are not just about ingredients. The consistency of the meal is also important – whether it is liquefied, pureed, soft, chopped or otherwise mechanically altered. Nursing home meals are regulated by strict guidelines – for example, the number of hours that should lapse between breakfast and the evening meal. This inflexibility prevents homes from offering late breakfasts to those who don't rise early. Most rules, however, reflect simple common sense. Sanitary conditions must be maintained in the kitchens, and all refuse must be properly disposed of.

Most homes do not employ their own registered dietician, but for the past 15 years, our facility has hired one to supervise our food preparation, expanding to hire another when we opened a subacute program. Seriously ill patients are helped by being provided with clinical dietetic services. Although most homes can't count on a full-time dietician, they do usually use their consultancy services, and purchase menus for all of the special diets that need to be followed, including diets low in salt and so on.

The provision of therapeutic meals to those who need them is required by law. The case study below clearly illustrates the vast difference that a proper diet can make to the quality of life of a nursing home resident.

Case Study

The importance of diet to nursing home resident's general health and well being is often under-estimated. Selena Leare, resident of Hot Springs Nursing home knows that it should not be! Three years ago, when Selena came to live at Hot Springs at the age of 85, she was seriously underweight. For years, she'd been having difficulty digesting her food. As a sufferer of osteoporosis,

Selena knew how important it was to have a diet high in calcium, and she was always very careful to drink plenty of milk and eat lots of cheese, together with hearty portions of fresh vegetables and lean meat. Selena's diet seemed so healthy, that her son and daughter wondered why she couldn't maintain a healthy body weight. By the time she moved from her own home to a nursing home, she was more than thirty pounds underweight, and suffered from chronic cramping, nausea and persistent diarrhea.

After meeting with the consultant dietician who served the facility, Selena's only regret was that she hadn't sought professional help earlier. It didn't take long for him to realize that Selena was lactose intolerant. The condition had caused her few problems when she was younger – and before she started consuming so much dairy produce – but old age, and changes in her eating habits had brought it to the fore. Gareth worked closely with Selena and the kitchen staff of Hot Springs to put together a menu plan that was both healthy and palatable. He recommended non-dairy sources of calcium, including enriched orange juice for breakfast and dark green leaf vegetables. Selena's system was quick to respond to the new regimen, and within three months she had returned to the right weight for her height and build. At 88, Selena is one of Hot Springs' most active residents. She has to be careful to avoid falls because of her brittle bones, but she takes part in group outings and activities with enthusiasm, and now that she knows which foodstuffs to avoid, is proud to boast of her "cast-iron digestion".

Selena's case is yet another example of how investment in specialist professionals costs everyone less money in the long-term. Quite apart from saving Selena what may have been years of discomfort and pain, Gareth's menu plan transformed her from a dangerously thin, persistently sickly old woman to a robust, active senior citizen. Selena needs few medications to keep her well. Without the help of a dietician, she would quickly have become dehydrated, in need of intravenous feeding, and vulnerable to the many conditions that affect the bed-ridden – pressure sores, muscle wastage, urinary tract infections and more.

Case Study

The case study I report below refers to a resident who stayed for some time in my nursing home, St. Luke's. Her daughter was kind enough to contribute her story to this book.

My mother was a patient at St. Luke's Subacute Hospital. We chose St. Luke's because my mother, who was in a coma following a stroke, was in need of special care. She needed ventilator assistance to breath, and daily doses of insulin. She was unable to eat, and had to be fed intravenously. She'd developed secondary problems in hospital and needed to be carefully watched at all times. When she was discharged from the hospital, I was afraid that the care she received just wouldn't be enough, but I was reassured when I met the staff who were there to take care of her. Shortly after her admission to the nursing home, I met with the clinical dietician, the director of nurses, the social worker and a respiratory specialist. Although I'd thought that my mother's biggest difficulty were her pulmonary problems, they warned me about the dangers of malnutrition, and the possibility of complications from inefficient metabolism of her food. The dietician explained that she'd done an assessment to discover what her energy and protein requirements were, and the director of nurses described how good airway management and nursing skills can help to reduce breathing difficulties. For the first time, I began to hope that Mom might be able to live without a ventilator. The dietician recommended a change in Mom's diet in order in minimize the production of carbon dioxide and maintain her blood sugar levels – now she was provided the 100% of her calorie and protein needs, as well as adequate minerals and vitamins. Gradually, the respiratory therapist was able to take her off the ventilator. Before long, she'd gained four pounds, her albumin had increased and she began to wake up. Although there were a number of minor crises, she improved to the point whereby I could take her to an institution close to my home, enabling me to visit more frequently.

The typical nursing home's director of food service is a high school graduate familiar with the ins and outs of kitchen work. He or she is responsible for ensuring the freshness of food, ordering new supplies in a timely manner, keeping an eye on the quality of ingredients, and so on. In homes with their own dietician, he or she works beneath their charge – otherwise, the consultant dietician visits once a month or provides advice from outside. The food service director is also responsible for meeting families and residents to discuss ways in which the individual requests and needs of each resident can be met within the limits of their dietary requirements. Food service directors are required to hold at least a high school diploma, and to graduate from a 36-hour dietetic training program approved by the state.

Cooks prepare food according to the instructions handed down by the dietician and food service supervisor. Generally, different cooks take care of the various courses of each meal. I have to say that cooks are among the unsung heroes of the healthcare system. Trained on the job, they are usually the first employees to arrive every morning. A good cook's strength lies in being able to produce a variety of meals in large quantities, that will prove palatable to the often multi-ethnic standards of modern nursing homes. Over the years, cooks develop the skills necessary for producing meals that taste good even though they may have no salt, and are made of cheap ingredients. Even textureless, pureed meals and mechanically altered foods have to be prepared in such a way as to be pleasant to eat.

Kitchen helpers are on hand in every facility's food preparation area to take care of washing dishes, kitchen hygiene, general maintenance and the delivery of the residents' food trays to the nursing floor, where the nurses' aides give the meal to each resident in their room, hallway or dining room. Nurses' aides are responsible for recovering the meal trays when the residents have finished eating. Many cooks begin working in nursing homes as kitchen helpers, and gradually learn their trade from more experienced kitchen staff.

Activity Services

A good nursing home is not just a place for the ill and dying. It is also a place to live, and pleasure is a crucial aspect of life. Organized activities are important for elderly residents who may lack motivation to do things by themselves – and they also help to keep minds alert, introduce people to one another and boost morale. Various staff members take care of this important aspect of healthcare.

Recreational therapists provide treatment services and recreational activities to nursing home residents, using a range of techniques to treat or maintain the physical, mental, and emotional well being of clients, including arts and crafts, contact with animals, sports, games, dance and movement, drama, music, and community outings. Involvement in activities on a regular basis helps to keep depression, stress and anxiety to a minimum, while playing an important part in restoring motor function, the power of reason and general confidence. Recreational therapists organize specific activities to help people with specific needs, consulting with nursing staff, psychologists and physical therapists. Therapists also observe and document patients' participation, reactions and progress. A minority of homes employs recreational therapists, as they are not required by federal or state regulations. Activity directors, who organize activities for residents, are required by law, but recreational therapists do much more than just schedule and conduct activities, consulting with nursing staff, psychologists and physical therapists, as well as observing and documenting patients' participation, reactions and progress.

Case Study

I can't stress strongly enough the importance of recreational therapy. After many years of working in the nursing home industry, I've seen the huge difference they can make to residents' lives.

One patient of ours, Linda, stayed in her room and refused to take part in any activities. Although she was within her rights, we could see that this isolation wasn't doing her any good. Our recreational therapist visited her every day – often twice – and a friendship developed. With encouragement, Linda gradually felt able to spend time with other residents. Now, she enjoys exercise classes, music therapy and interacting with her peers. From being unable to walk, she has become mobile and will soon be transferred to the community for more independent living.

Kim was ventilator-dependent when she came to the facility. She was unable to speak and take part in activities. Our recreational therapist began sensory stimulation and music therapy with her and over the last few months Kim has made wonderful progress. She is now breathing by herself. She sings in music class, and takes special exercises to help her with her right side paralysis.

Sun, who is from Korea, came to our facility for rehabilitation services after having suffered a stroke. She had become paraplegic and was depressed. With physical therapy, her upper body strength improved, and with some encouragement she began attending music classes and other activities. Her self-esteem has improved enormously, and she has made friends.

One service that therapists, including recreational therapists, provide is that of grief therapy. You might say that losing loved ones to death is an "occupational hazard" of being elderly. Of course, we all know that death is inevitable, and that death after a long life is not a bad thing, but part of the natural cycle of existence. Those of us who are religious may believe in an afterlife or in reincarnation. None of this makes the pain of loss easy to bear. Grieving affects the psychological well being of the bereaved, and can also have profound implications for their physical health. Recreational therapy can be one way to help start remembering instead of mourning.

Case Study

Mrs. Johns, at 73, had lived with her husband in the same nursing home for eight years until his death. As soon as the funeral was over, she insisted on moving to live in our nursing home. She didn't want to be surrounded by memories, and hoped to get on with her life. She never gave herself any time to mourn her loss. However, from the moment she was admitted, she suffered from chronic sleeplessness and depression. Working together with her, our staff helped her to speak about her grief and her fear of the future. She spoke of other people whom she had lost, of how much she missed them, and of her continuing need to be loved and have friends. Little by little she adjusted to her losses and began to be able to take part in activities with other residents. She had been thinking of moving again, but as she made new friends and started being able to sleep through the night, her depression lifted and she decided to stay.

Depression in the elderly can often be helped by assisting them in finding new and old interests and talents that can be modified to their new abilities. Sometimes, these talents can be used in co-operation with others.

The presence of an activity director in every nursing home is required by the law. The main function of this nursing home employee is to provide activities for the residents throughout the day. In order to qualify for the position, employees must complete a 36-hour state approved course in activities. Activity directors generally devise monthly activity calendars, which incorporate those activities requested by the residents. These provide opportunities for residents to become involved in meaningful activities, and consequently it is vital that the activity leader be interested in making the program interesting and appealing. Sadly, many nursing home administrators do not recognize the important contribution of an activity to the welfare of elderly residents. Many nursing homes allocate a token budget of $100 per month in costs, making the task of providing a good program impossible for even the most enterprising activity director.

Good nursing homes appoint someone to act as director of volunteers – but most do not and instead leave these duties to the activity director or to the administration of a local religious group. Nursing homes that manage to develop and sustain a volunteer program quickly recognize the extent to which it enhances their service. However, federal and state government do not require viable volunteer programs and consequently management is generally reluctant to expend time and money on such a program. The wonderful aspect of volunteer work in nursing homes is that it makes them an integral part of the local community, rather than isolated warehouses for the elderly.

Rehabilitation Department

Not every home has its own in-house rehabilitation department, with those that don't contracting out for services including physical, speech and occupational therapy as needed or according to the physician's instructions.

Physical therapists provide services designed to help improve residents' mobility as well as restore the function of worn limbs and relieve the pain of those patients suffering from conditions such as arthritis or fractured bones. A treatment plan is developed for each resident, with the aim of making him or her as mobile and self-sufficient as possible. Treatments include exercises to improve balance, coordination, endurance and strength as well as massage, electrical stimulation and more. Physical therapists also teach residents how to use crutches, prostheses (artificial limbs) and wheelchairs.

Case Study

Timothy Travers had to have his left leg amputated when he developed diabetes related gangrene. On being released from hospital, he entered the subacute ward at the Pope John Paul Nursing Home near Boston. Although he was expected to make a good recovery, and be able to return home, it was important that he be closely monitored as his wound healed. Timothy was still relatively young at 62, and there was every reason to hope that he would be able to acquire an excellent degree of mobility. Although he had just undergone an amputation and was dealing with both the physical and the psychological fall-out from the operation, Timothy brought with him a very positive attitude. He benefited from the help of the consultant dietician, who counseled him as to how he might tailor his diet to control his diabetes, preventing further amputations, and from the psychologist, who talked him through the issues usually faced by people in his situation, but he was especially helped by the in-house physical therapist, Jennifer Alexander.

The most obvious difficulty facing Tim was that of having to learn how to walk with an artificial leg – but diabetes also affects blood vessels, nerves and energy transportation, as it deprives muscles and other soft tissues of nutrients and oxygen. If Tim were to maintain a reasonable level of mobility, and avoid further amputations, he would have to be very careful. Tim was in subacute care for a total of five months, during which time he learned how to walk with his new prosthetic limb. With the help of the dietician, he lost weight and started to follow a healthier eating plan. Despite the pain and discomfort he suffered in the process of relearning how to walk, Tim had one thing going for him for as long as he was in subacute care – he saw his physical therapist every day, and was cajoled, encouraged and even bullied into following an exercise program. He made an excellent recovery, and, when the time came, was able to walk out of the nursing home and into his wife's car. Exercise and extra care can't stop outside the nursing home, however, and Jenny had supplied him with an exercise plan to follow, minimizing the risk of a further onset of gangrene and another amputation.

Occupational therapists help people to improve their ability to perform tasks in their daily living and working environments by working towards maximizing their motor functions and reasoning abilities, and helping to compensate for permanent loss of function in certain areas. Therapy methods range from physical exercises to exercises intended to improve visual function or hand to eye coordination. Recording the residents' activities and progress is an important aspect of the job.

Case Study

Alison Hilary had diabetes-related gangrene that resulted in the amputation of both of her legs above the knee. She made a reasonably good recovery, but at 78 years of age wasn't strong enough to start walking again, and had to become wheelchair bound. Her doctor and family both felt that there was no need for her to remain in a nursing home indefinitely – as long as she could master the art of managing her daily routine from a chair. Although she was obviously distressed by the recent amputation, Alison had a positive approach to her situation, and welcomed the help of occupational therapist Christianne Moore.

Everything changes when one is in a wheelchair. Suddenly, steps are obstacles, kitchen counters are too high and, until you learn how to manage the chair, getting washed and dressed can be a logistical nightmare. While she remained in the home, Alison worked with Christianne three times a week perfecting techniques to maximize her independence. In the meantime, her son Ian had an annex to his house made wheelchair friendly, so that Alison could move in when she was ready. With a lot of determination, Alison was able to leave the nursing home after seeing her occupational therapist for two and a half months, and even manages to cook and serve meals in her adapted kitchen.

Certain medical conditions, such as strokes, can leave people with difficulty speaking. Speech therapists help to retrain residents to communicate verbally by working with their language, cognitive ability, swallowing and other related issues. A care-plan packaged to each resident's needs is developed. Recovering the power of speech is vital in enabling stroke victims and others to become re-integrated into society – the inability to communicate properly causes more than just practical difficulties, it also isolates and stigmatizes the sufferer.

Medical Services

Medical services are provided to nursing home residents by specialists in a range of areas, who work together with the attending family physician. These include a psychiatrist, a dentist and other physicians with specialties including cardiologists, dermatologists, infectious disease specialists, internists, neurologists, orthopedists, pain management experts, urologists, podiatrists and psychologists. Most nursing homes have a medical director who is affiliated with them on a part-time basis, and usually visits just once a month to review the services and attend meetings. He or she must provide services on a consultancy basis, and usually acts as the attending physician for many residents, implementing nursing home admission, transfers and discharges, overseeing infection control, the use of restraints and the duties of the non-physician healthcare workers (nursing and others). The medical director must also generate policies with respect to accidents, extra services such as laboratory testing, the use and release of clinical information and overall quality of care. He or she should also coordinate medical care in the nursing home, monitor and ensure the implementation of resident care policies and oversee physician services. If the medical director identifies, or receives a report of, possible inadequate medical care, including inappropriate drug treatments, the situation must be evaluated, and steps taken to correct the problem. Most nursing homes have a medical director who is affiliated with them on a part-time basis, and visits just once a month to review the services and attend meetings.

All residents ideally have an attending physician who first becomes involved with the home when he or she writes a recommendation that their patient be admitted. From then on, the resident remains beneath this physician's care. He or she participates in assessment and care planning, notes changes in medical status and provides consultation and treatment services as necessary. The physician should implement treatments designed to ensure the highest possible standard of living for the resident, ordering specialist treatments when and if necessary. In many cases, a resident's attending physician is also the home's medical director.

A large percentage of nursing home residents suffer from mental illness – most commonly either Alzheimer's or depression. Nurses and other medical staff, competent as they may be, are not always able to diagnose and treat mental illness properly. For example, Prozac, a drug commonly used to treat depression, can cause weight loss in the elderly. A psychiatrist knows this, and can choose a more apt medication to treat this condition in a vulnerable patient. It's also important to understand the exact reason for violent, irrational behavior in the demented. For example, if a patient with Alzheimer's develops a urinary tract infection, he or she may not be able to tell nurses what's wrong, and react instead, by becoming angry and violent. Using tranquilizers in these cases just won't work. The state of mental health of a nursing home's residents can also be enhanced by ensuring that a psychologist is available to provide advice and consultation. Psychologists study the human mind and human behavior. In the context of a nursing home, they provide mental healthcare to residents who may have difficulty adjusting, rather that to those who are suffering from a mental illness. Geropsychologists deal with the special problems that face elderly people. Another medical service essential to the care of the elderly is dentistry. Every nursing facility has a professional relationship with a dentist who oversees residents' dental care with checkups and treatment as necessary. Unfortunately, this service is often overlooked and many nursing home residents never obtain regular dental services. Medicare will only cover the costs involved if a medical physician is called upon to intervene.

Nursing homes contract with a licensed pharmacist for consultancy services with regard to the provision of pharmacy services in the facility. The pharmacist also establishes a system of records of each time drugs have been purchased and administered. An account of all controlled drugs is maintained. Pharmacists should also review the medication received by all residents on a monthly basis, to ensure that the various drugs they are taking are mutually compatible. Any irregularities should be reported to the attending physician, the director of nursing and the medical director of the facility. The pharmacist is also responsible for ensuring that drugs are properly stored under lock and key and kept at an appropriate temperature.

Well- managed nursing homes always ensure that they have an up-to-date list of local medical specialists whom they can contact for residents suffering from conditions beyond the scope of the regular staff. When the need occurs, they employ their services to help with diagnosis and the development of a treatment plan.

Each nursing home must make arrangements for whatever diagnostic services are necessary, including radiology (x-ray) and laboratory services. These must be provided by a certified Medicare provider, and should be used for the diagnosis, treatment, prevention or assessment of the medical condition of the resident. All laboratory and other reports should be filed in the medical record of the resident in question.

Some medical conditions call for specialist help. When this occurs, consultants are brought in to assist with diagnosis and developing a treatment plan.

The role of the medical record clerk and his or her assistant is, in some ways, not unlike that of the librarian or archivist. The great difference is, of course, that if a book goes missing from a library, the client has to pay to replace it. If a resident's records go missing, he or she may pay a much more significant price. Each nursing home's medical records department is responsible for having a medical record of each resident, which must be complete, accurately documented, readily accessible and systematically organized. The medical record should contain accurate, reliable documentation pertaining to the actual experience of the resident. This record shows their health status, the care plans that have been devised for them, and details about their response to treatment, change in condition and changes in treatment. When care plan goals are changed, the medical record should document this shift. Clinical records should be kept for at least five years from the date of discharge or transferred when a resident moves to another organization. Medical record supervisors are responsible for safeguarding clinical record information against loss, destruction or unauthorized use. The record is a confidential document that should only be released when the resident is transferred to another healthcare institution, when the law requires it or at the resident's request.

Social Services

Only nursing homes with 120 or more beds are required to hire a social worker, who should hold at least an undergraduate degree in social work or a related field, as well as one year of supervised social work experience in a healthcare setting working directly with individuals. Smaller homes use outside services, usually designating a specific employee to make the arrangements when necessary. A social worker's job is to help people to function as well as they can in their given environment, and to intervene in solving personal, family or relational problems. Working directly with the residents, they help them to identify concerns, consider solutions and find answers to problems. Social workers may also organize support groups for the families of people with Alzheimer's or other diseases.

Case Study

Janice Clark was desperately unhappy in Aurora Nursing home. Years earlier, she'd had a bitter disagreement with her daughter, from whom she was now completely estranged. Her husband had died five years before, and she had few friends. Reluctant to contact her daughter after such a long time, she was resigned to staying alone and lonely. Although the home was well run and pleasant, many of the other residents suffered from Alzheimer's to varying degrees and it wasn't easy finding someone to talk to. Nursing Director Kitty Reynolds asked the home's visiting social worker Alan James to look at Janice's case. She knew that Janice would be a lot happier if she had someone to talk to once in a while, and that happier patients are easier to take care of, and more likely to respond to treatment. The situation was really very straightforward – Janice was lonely. Alan talked her through the argument that she'd had with her daughter many years ago, and persuaded Janice to get in touch. Mary was a stockbroker in New York now, and had no idea that her mother had gone to live in a nursing home. Contact was established, and now she visits from time to time and keeps in touch by letter and telephone. They'll never be the best of friends, but this is an immense improvement. Alan also got in touch with a local volunteer organization that matches lonely nursing home residents with people in the community who are willing to visit them and keep them company from time to time. Janice's new visitor was a big success. A woman in her early fifties, her children had recently left home, and she had some time on her hands. Janice's loneliness has retreated and she has become easier to care for and generally more content. Alan often has to deal with infinitely more complex situations – this was one case where the solution to the problem was quite easy to find!

The Physical Environment

The physical environment of the nursing home is the responsibility of the housekeeping, laundry and maintenance services of the hospital. Are you ever surprised by just how much work it is keeping your own home clean and tidy – not to mention keeping up with house electrical maintenance, plumbing, appliances, air conditioning and central heating, pest control, landscaping …? Imagine how much more work goes into keeping a nursing facility in order! Too many nursing homes are not kept properly clean, forcing residents to live – and nursing staff to work – in a foul-smelling environment. A full cleaning and maintenance staff is very important, and their contribution to the nursing home is recognized in the laws of the United States.

The housekeeping supervisor is the person who coordinates the efforts of all of the domestic staff – usually while also actively participating in the work, making sure that supplies are ordered on time and that cleaning and other maintenance work is done efficiently and thoroughly. Housekeepers are employees who take care of the crucial task of keeping things clean and orderly, cleaning bedrooms, bathrooms and floors throughout the hospital. No nursing home could function without them! A janitor should also always be on hand to take care of the heavy work of cleaning windows, floors and equipment. He may also be able to provide basic help with electrical matters, paintwork and more.

Most nursing homes provide their own laundry services, washing items such as bed linens, blankets and residents' personal clothes items. Unfortunately, the laundry service is often also a major source of complaints from residents and their families, and an expensive liability for the home, as items are frequently lost, stolen or misplaced. The laundry service must also handle, store, process and transport in such a manner as to prevent the spread of infection. Soiled linens and clothes are handled in containers to minimize the release of airborne contaminants and prevent the workers' exposure to any waste material. Soiled and clean linens and clothes must always be kept carefully separated to prevent any cross-contamination. Nursing homes that provide laundry services hire a laundry supervisor, who both works, and co-ordinates the efforts of other staff – and they have a lot to take care of! Every home must count with at least three full changes of linen, and laundry workers are fully occupied keeping a set clean and dry at all times.

Nursing homes also need to be able to count on someone experienced in the maintenance of buildings, with skills to diagnose and fix simple problems, including electrical and plumbing malfunctions. The maintenance worker should also be able to paint, do basic woodwork, and oversee the heating and air conditioning systems. Maintenance, like other aspects of running a nursing home, is subject to multiple rules and regulations, all of which are necessary to ensure the health and safety of the residents. Perhaps the most important of the maintenance worker's responsibilities is that of protecting the home and its residents from fire. All nursing homes are required to meet the minimum standards set out in the 1985 edition of the Life Safety Code of National Fire Protection.

Another major issue is that of maintaining the emergency power system so as to supply power for all entrances and exits in the case of a shortage, equipment to maintain fire detection, alarms and extinguishing systems and life support systems. Maintenance is also required to keep mechanical, electrical and patient care equipment in safe operating condition – from refrigerators and freezers to laundry equipment. A call system should also maintained at the nursing station to receive calls from residents through a communication system, while toilet and bathing facilities must be kept working, with proper lighting and ventilation. In order to minimize breakdowns, a preventative maintenance program should be followed. Another issue that is the responsibility of maintenance is that of ensuring that the facility is free of common household pests such as cockroaches, flies and mice at all times.

Inspection

While they aren't employees of nursing homes, inspectors play a large role in their functioning. The Centers for Medicare and Medicaid Services (CMS) is the federal agency that watches over homes. It requires the state to conduct surprise inspections of homes between every 9 to 15 months, and states usually assign their Department of Health to the task. The survey is conducted by a multidisciplinary team of professionals, at least one of whom must be a registered nurse. Surveyors are obliged to complete a training and testing program in survey and certification techniques approved by federal government. The purpose of inspections is to ensure that homes meet the quality and performance standards met by Medicare. Homes that are determined not to meet these standards are inspected more frequently. Inspectors also investigate complaints when they arise, and interview staff, residents and residents' families to assess the quality of the service provided as well as overlooking the medical records. Inspectors with specialized training include fire safety inspectors. The inspection process can best be described by calling it a "negative" process. That means that inspectors only look for what is wrong with a home – a report will never contain details about what the home is doing well. The inspectors' job is to isolate problems and issue citations, which they do by using the over 500 pre-defined criteria they are supplied with. Despite attempts at regularization, considerable discrepancies can be found from one state to the next, with some states citing more than half of all homes as in serious breach of the rules, and some citing only a few. The problem lies in the language of the law, which defines issues in general terms open to personal interpretation. These inconsistencies are worrying – to what extent can we trust the system to tell us how efficient our nursing homes really are? Too often, homes that are genuinely providing the best service they can with the funding they have become caught in a bureaucratic war between state and federal government, which invariably have differing views as to the enforcement of the regulations. Further problems arise when different homes receive very different treatment, with one institution cited for a violation for a problem that might barely get a mention elsewhere. The nursing home's best defense against being cited for a deficiency is its paperwork. In most cases, if the paperwork indicates that residents are seen on a regular basis, the inspectors are content that they are. The need to generate more and more paperwork to impress visiting inspectors, however, takes nurses away from their real responsibilities – caring for the residents.

Homes that are found to be gravely deficient face a range of penalties, usually a fine, but sometimes closure. While penalties are often necessary, these actions are counterproductive in terms of improving nursing care. America already lacks sufficient homes for its elderly, and money taken from the institutions ultimately affects its elderly residents in terms of a reduction of the quality of service.

The Nursing Home Residents

It can be easy to lose sight of the fact that nursing homes are supposed to be about the care of individual people, and not just machines that work according to the federal and state regulations. But what are the basic rules that govern the treatment of residents at the hands of nursing and other staff? The federal government has, in fact, developed a tool that each nursing home can use to assess, on admission and periodically thereafter, each resident's functional capacity and treatment needs. Once the needs have been identified, the nursing department puts together a care plan tailored for the individual in question. This plan provides the basis for the identification of all future needs, and is an important tool in ensuring that the requisite care is documented. The criteria that must be dealt with are the following:

- Identification and demographic information
- Customary routine
- Cognitive patterns
- Communication
- Vision
- Mood and behavior patterns
- Psychosocial well being
- Physical functioning and structural problems
- Continence
- Disease diagnoses and health conditions
- Dental and nutritional status
- Skin condition
- Activity pursuit
- Medications
- Special treatments and procedures
- Discharge potential
- Documentation of summary information regarding the additional assessment performed through the resident assessment protocols
- Documentation of participation in assessment

The assessment, whether on the resident's admission or thereafter, should include direct observation and communication with the resident, as well as with the licensed and non-licensed staff members on all shifts. A comprehensive assessment should be conducted within 14 days of admission, or after a significant change in the person's physical or mental state. A full assessment should be conducted every year, and a quarterly review assessment every 3 months. The law requires that certain data from the assessment be automated and certified as true by the nursing home in question.

False materials or statements make the home liable to be tried in a civil court, and penalized to the tune of at least $1000. Comprehensive assessments are intended to provide the foundation for a comprehensive care plan for each resident, with specific objectives and timetables designed to meet all of the person's medical, physical and other needs. Care plans should include the services provided to attain or maintain the resident's highest practicable physical, mental, and psychosocial well being while respecting the residents' right to refuse treatment. Care plans should be prepared by an interdisciplinary team, including the physician, a registered nurse responsible for the resident and other relevant staff members as well as the resident and his or her family.

It all sounds impressive, doesn't it? The problem is this; if a nursing home provides documentation suggesting that it has provided proper care, in most cases the inspectors will assume that it has indeed done so. If it does not, then it is assumed to have neglected the patient. The issue that is questioned is always that of documentation and not that of resident health and well being. Care that was not documented is not considered to have taken place, placing the emphasis on paperwork and not resident well being.

CHAPTER FOUR: THE LOOMING CRISIS [8]

In the modern world, thanks to the dramatic pharmacological and medical developments we have seen in recent decades, more and more people are surviving to advanced ages. However, not all of our senior citizens enjoy good health in their declining years, and many need full-time nursing care – not necessarily for a specific complaint, but rather for the debilitating condition called aging. Others, although physically well, do not retain their grasp on reality, and may become confused, demented and even dangerous to themselves or others. These are not pleasant facts to dwell upon, but it is important to remember that we all grow old! In caring properly for today's senior citizens, we lay the groundwork for the humane treatment of tomorrow's elderly among whom we must count ourselves. There is a well-known folktale in Europe that is particularly apt here.

Once upon a time, there lived a couple and their little boy together with the husband's elderly father. This poor man was very, very old, and was no longer able to care for himself. When he ate, his hands trembled, and his son and daughter in law pointed at him and laughed, calling him stupid. His memory was not what it used to be, either, and when he forgot things, they would ridicule him. Instead of taking care of him, as a dutiful family would, they tied him to a chair and left him in a corner of their house. At mealtimes, instead of inviting him to eat at table with the family, they gave him a little trough to eat from, as if he were a pig rather than a man.

One day, the parents of the little boy found him playing very earnestly with a small set of tools and some pieces of wood.

---

[8] In this chapter, use has been made of the information provided in Susan Eaton's (Institute for Work and Employment Research, Sloan School of Management, MIT and Radcliffe Public Policy Center, Radcliffe Institute for Advanced Studies) Beyond 'unloving care:' inking human resource management and patient care quality in nursing homes." *International Journal of Human Resource Management,* Volume 22, No. 3. June: 591-616.

"What are you doing?" they asked.

"I'm making a little trough for you to eat from, when you are old," the little boy answered, "so that I can watch and laugh at you as you eat."

At this, the parents were very shocked. They hadn't even stopped to ask themselves if their behavior towards the old man was correct or not. From then on, they were always careful to treat him with respect – especially in front of their little boy!

The percentage of elderly people in the population is increasing, and will continue to increase in the decades to come. Within the next quarter century, the number of American citizens of sixty five years of age or more will rise to around 50 million from the 34 million of today. The age group that currently exhausts most healthcare funding is the group aged 85 and more, and this sector of society has been predicted to rise by 3.4 million by the year 2020, to a total of 6.7 million. These changes in population are not just statistical. They will create the need for more intensive care in nursing homes all over the nation, along with a corresponding increase in demand for medical resources, and an increased need of qualified nursing and other professional medical staff.

The revolution that introduced more females than ever before to the workplace has also reduced the number of women available to provide unpaid nursing care to elderly relatives – until quite recently, a traditional feminine role. Progress in medical treatment, surgical techniques and the pharmaceutical area means that many patients now survive to an advanced age, by which stage they need constant care. For all of these reasons nursing homes will become more and more important in the United States.

Case Study: A Glimpse at the Future

What does the future hold for nursing care facilities in the United States? One hopes that the reality will not be as bleak as the one I depict. However, we are on course for creating a terrible future for ourselves. Assuming that nothing is done to redress this, let's take a look:

August 15th, 2035

Richard Sneggley, aged 79, was recently forced by his diminishing levels of mobility to move to Ashford Nursing Home – the same home where his mother had moved to live thirty years earlier. As he was wheeled through the front door, he noticed that it had not changed very much. In fact, the new paint job seemed to be the only real difference.

As a young man, Richard worked for Microsoft, and had made regular healthcare payments towards the future. The income these provide are not enough to pay the nursing home the substantial sum it requires to care for Richard, and he is also in receipt of Medicare payments. Despite repeated calls from the industry for reform, Medicare and Medicaid have remained essentially as they were long before Richard even thought of retiring.

The population of the United States has a higher percentage of senior citizens than ever before. The average age of death has risen considerably, thanks to developments in medicine, but these extra years seem to many more like a sentence than a gift. Nursing homes still operate with one nurses' aide caring for every eight residents, and a charge and medication nurse overseeing their efforts.

Meals are no longer prepared in the nursing home. Ashford Nursing Home buys in pre-prepared meals from a catering agency which provides food for a wide range of facilities – this became the most efficient and cost-effective way of providing food for the elderly. The kitchen is closely inspected, and directed by a dietician who uses approved menus from the Department of Health. There are no more complaints about the preparation and delivery of food – but there are complaints from residents, who don't get what they asked for, and don't like the food. All the nursing home administration can say is that they have no control over the kitchen and preparation, that the kitchen is certified and inspected by the Department of Health, and that it meets all health and regulatory standards.

When Richard moved to Ashford Nursing home, he was still able to walk, although he did need some help getting in and out of bed. He was assured that he would be kept clean and out of bed, and that he could participate in the home's activities both in the morning and in the afternoon. He would be consulted about his treatment plan, would see the doctor every month and should only call the charge nurse if he needed anything.

"You are responsible for bringing your needs to the attention of the nursing staff," he was warned.

The Crisis in America's Nursing Homes

When Richard was put in bed, he was fitted with small, compact monitoring devices that would send data about his vital signs and monitor his movements. He also noticed a small computer camera in his room – the technology was out of date, but functional. Richard would be observed at the central observation station, saving staff from having to actually check on him in person. Unless Richard's monitors or the camera revealed signs of distress, he would have no contact with nursing staff for hours at a time. Probes were placed in his bed to detect wetness, and whether Richard needed a diaper or bed linen changed – although it still takes about two hours to get around to changing a wet patient, just as it did more than three decades earlier. In the best-supervised homes, the interval is about 20 minutes.

Richard does not have to worry about his basic needs. His food is prepared in a centralized, approved kitchen with menus planned by dieticians. He is constantly monitored and if something goes wrong, attended to. Activities are available both in the morning and the afternoon. What more could he want?

Richard's usual contact with his nurses' aide is when she comes around with the medication cart. This dispenses his medicine directly into a cup, which is then handed to him. Years ago, when Richard's mother was in the same home, the nurse would bring the medication cart to her room, and talk to her while dispensing the medicine and checking to see if her patient had every she needed. Now the procedure takes seconds, and few words are exchanged.

Another big change is the fact that all the nurses' aides and nurses wear full protective gear, including face masks, gowns, gloves and shoe covers. In the three months of Richard's stay, he has never been touched by a human hand. Nor has he ever seen the faces of the nursing staff who care for him. When he asked why, he was told that these precautions were to prevent the spread of infection to either staff or residents.

The United States, together with the European Union and Japan, leads the world in medical technology. But tuberculosis is a major problem among America's poor and elderly, and the conditions in Medicare supported nursing homes are an embarrassment to the nation. Help is hard to find. Nursing homes are less attractive in the eyes of many, having a work force largely composed of ethnic minorities and recent immigrants. Working in a nursing home is considered the least desirable of all possible occupations in the America of 2035.

Wealthy senior citizens pay huge sums for adequate care in expensive private homes, but they are in a minority. Most nursing-home bound elders are supported, at least in part, by Medicare. Payments have increased slowly over the years, at a rate consistently lower than the rate of inflation.

Public support for euthanasia has grown so strong, that congress will shortly be voting on a bill to make it legal in a wide range of circumstances. Families of nursing home residents, distressed by the conditions in which their loved ones live, often feel that they would be better off "out of their misery". Ironically, much of this misery is caused less by age, and more by the serious lack of funding and staffing. American citizens approaching old age are encouraged to draw up legal documents defining the circumstances under which they should be "allowed to die." Euthanasia is a growth industry.

Richard is slightly muddled at times – especially early in the morning, or if he has forgotten to take his medication. A strong opponent of euthanasia, he always refused to sign any document allowing medical staff or family to take important decisions about his future without his consent. If he becomes more confused, however, it's possible that his son could become his legal guardian, and give his permission to have medication and even food and water withdrawn.

With proper care, Richard would still be able to live an active, productive life for several years. But, as things are, this is not possible, and he will be lucky if he avoids being "put out of his misery" by a family and nursing staff that have convinced themselves that they would be doing the right thing.

The Privatization of Nursing Homes

Since 1970, ever-smaller numbers of nursing homes have been run by private individuals. Little by little, these have been taken over by large corporations until now only a handful are run on a smaller, more personal scale – my many years as an administrator and supervisor of nursing homes have given me an inside view on how they have changed, and how they are organized and maintained. According to Susan Eaton, of the Sloan School of Management, there are now more than one and half million people living in 17,300 American nursing homes, cared for by almost 2 million employees. She states that the population of nursing homes will double in 25 years, and triple in 35 as members of the so-called "baby boom generation" become elderly. "Baby boomers" – those born between 1946 and 1964, many of whom are now nearing retirement age – reached adulthood in an era in which it was reasonable to expect government supported healthcare to improve or, at least, not to decline in quality and coverage. Because of their faith that the nation would provide for them in their old age – from the taxes that they have paid throughout a lifetime of work – many of this generation have not saved enough to pay for the nursing care that they may require. According to a recent study [9], the median amount of assets set aside by a typical baby boomer is $30,000 – considerably less than the cost of a year in a nursing facility when the average length of stay is 2.3 years. Many of this generation, having secured comfortable livings throughout their working years, will end their lives in poverty unless the crisis situation is addressed.

Although public discussion of the nursing home crisis began in the mid 1980s [10], few of the issues raised then have been addressed. In 1986, Charlene Harrington reported that the Institute of Medicine completed a study entitled "Improving the Quality of Care in Nursing Homes". At that point, attention was drawn to the rights of nursing home residents, the importance of staff and services, minimum training standards for nursing assistants, and means by which the quality of care in nursing homes should be monitored and reported. Then, the requirements for basic services were judged to be as follows: nursing homes should have one registered nurse as director of nursing, one registered nurse present in the home 8 hours per day, seven days per week and one licensed nurse, 24 hours per day; nursing assistants must have 75 hours training, and pass a competency exam; staffing must be sufficient to provide adequate care; there should be specialized rehabilitation, social, pharmaceutical, dietary, dental and activity services [11]. Many nursing homes still do not meet these basic requirements, despite public concern. Federal law requires that nursing homes "provide services and activities to attain or maintain the highest practicable

---

[9] From the National Center for Women and Retirement Research.

[10] Charlene Harrington, Ph.D., RN. *The Federal Nursing Home Survey and Regulation Process* Prepared for the U.S. Senate Special Committee on Aging, School of Nursing, University of California, San Francisco, 1998.

[11] Dan O'Sullivan, Press release, SEIU NURSE ALLIANCE, November 10, 2000.

physical, mental, and psychosocial well being of each resident." Many, however, fail to achieve federal health and safety standards.

Portrait of an Abusive Nursing Home – Time Magazine

Many nursing homes, despite their problems of understaffing and underfunding, go to great lengths to provide the best possible service for their residents. Some, however, maintain such poor conditions that they have been known to cause disability and even death. Here I quote an extract from a story widely circulated over the Internet, which was originally published on October 27th, 1997 by Time magazine. I wish I could tell you that things had changed significantly since that date. They have not.

Once she moved into Creekside Care Convalescent Hospital, it didn't take Bessie Seday long to realize that the promises made to her by the nursing home before she arrived had evaporated. "I couldn't get anybody's attention, starting on the fourth day," recalls the bed-bound 84-year-old. "You'd have your call light on for hours, but nobody came." What made her waiting more desolate was the near total deprivation of sunlight during her four months at Creekside. "It was a dungeon," she says. "I really would have liked to see the sunshine, but they never put us outside." Things only got worse when the sun set, and the staff ignored calls for help or pain-killers. "The screaming is what got to me the worst, the screaming when the lights went out," she says. "I couldn't fall asleep until 1 or 2 in the morning with all that screaming going on."

The article goes on to describe the scene that met Ms. Seday's daughter when she went to visit her mother:

"She was not turned and kept clean and dry, which led to the bedsores," Ann recalls. A bedsore on Bessie's left hip turned into a gaping wound that would not heal, despite repeated whirlpool baths. Creekside nurse Patricia Lloyd knew why: the special washing machine for cleaning dirty bedpans had broken down. "So we washed bedpans in the whirlpool," she says, "and then we'd put patients with big bedsores, like Bessie Seday, in there." Fixing Bessie's wound required repeated surgery, including the removal of her left buttock and part of her pelvis. "They were washing her," says Lesley Clement, her attorney, "in a damn cesspool."

Bessie Seday left the nursing institution, and moved to live elsewhere. However, as the original article makes more than clear, many senior citizens continue to live in such dire circumstances. After decades of ignorance, the American public has finally begun to realize what is going on:

Owing to the work of lawyers, investigators and politicians who have begun examining the causes of thousands of nursing-home deaths across the U.S., the grim details are emerging of an extensive, blood-chilling and for-profit pattern of neglect. In Chicago last week a 73-count indictment was returned against a hospice operator charged with milking Medicare and others of $28 million for services to the terminally ill that were never delivered. In Detroit a nursing home that was part of a chain whose owner was convicted of Medicaid fraud 17 years ago was cited again last year for bad hygiene, inattention to frail residents and incompetent staff. In Texas attorney general Dan Morales has filed 50 lawsuits against nursing homes this year for neglect and failure to medicate ... Palo Alto attorney Von Packard has studied the death certificates of all Californians who died in nursing homes from 1986 through 1993. More than 7% of them succumbed, at least in part, to utter neglect--lack of food or water, untreated bedsores or other generally preventable ailments. If in the rest of America's 1.6 million nursing-home residents are dying of questionable causes at the same rate as in California, it means that every year about 35,000 Americans are dying prematurely, or in unnecessary pain, or both. The investigations bear out something many Americans have suspected all along: in a recent survey published in the Journal of the American Geriatrics Society, 30% of those polled said they would rather perish than live in a nursing home. Packard, who has spent nearly two years tracking the data, says, "We believe thousands would have lived significantly longer had they been taken care of."

While abused elders are the real victims of nursing home understaffing and fraud, everybody has to pay:

Neglectful caregivers are preying not only on elderly residents but also on American taxpayers. More than $45 billion in government funds, mostly from Medicare and Medicaid, is pumped into nursing homes annually, an amount that comes to nearly 60% of the national tab for such eldercare. In order to pocket a larger slice of the federal stipend, many nursing homes—largely for-profit enterprises--provide a minimal level of care, if that ... Death comes to the elderly in many ways, including heart and lung failure, chronic disease and plain bad luck. But David Hoffman, an assistant U.S. attorney in Philadelphia, thought he spied something else at work last year, when he saw festering bedsores eating away the flesh of three residents in a local nursing home. He knew the home had been pocketing government money the residents were given to ensure good care, and he saw the bedsores as proof that they weren't getting it ... homes. She was startled to find 10 questionable causes of death listed on the first 30 she reviewed.

"They'd listed malnutrition, dehydration, bedsores and urinary-tract infections as causes of death," Swan says. "These nursing homes were killing people."

The TIME article highlights the fact that understaffing lies behind many, if not most, cases of nursing home abuse, and points to the problems that arise from insufficient staff numbers:

Many nursing homes have become dangerous places largely because they are understaffed--and underregulated. The Federal Government doesn't dictate staffing levels, and state efforts at regulating quality are meager. With 2 of every 3 dollars spent by nursing homes going to payrolls, the most tempting way to increase profits is to cut personnel ... Rhoda Johnson, Ila Swan's mother, lived at Creekside nearly two years, until July 1993. Her family alleged in a lawsuit that the nursing home essentially abandoned Johnson: she was often left lying in her own waste, hungry, cold, unfed and unturned. One day she complained to Swan that her hip hurt. With her sons' help, Swan lifted her mother out of the bed, pulled up her nightgown and collapsed in sobs. "She had this bedsore on her hip that was so deep," her daughter recalls, "that I could see the hip socket and leg bone moving inside the hole." Her bottom was bruised and caked with dried feces, which Swan peeled off with her fingers amid her tears. "I never had looked under the covers," she says. "I didn't think I had to." Johnson, now 98 and living in a Utah nursing home, doesn't talk much about her experience. "Creekside was mean to me," she says. "They didn't give me a drink, they yelled at me, they hurt me." She received a $775,000 settlement in May 1996.

Understaffing Issues

Nursing homes are already understaffed, and the wave of crisis has just begun to break. Working in a nursing home as a nurse or nurses' aide is difficult work, physically and emotionally. Elderly patients may need to be physically lifted and washed, and are often confused and distressed. Injuries, including repetitive strain injuries, are common among healthcare workers, who are more likely than almost any type of industrial worker to sustain a work-related illness or injury. Let's take a look at some of the figures revealed in a recent study.

What's the most dangerous job in America? Mining? Construction? Trucking? Working in a steel mill?

No. More dangerous than all of these—and fast becoming the most dangerous job in the United States—is nursing home work.

Ironically, nursing home work is also one of the fastest-growing jobs in America. While working conditions in many other industries have gradually improved over the last decade, nursing homes have become far more dangerous places to work. Caregivers suffer an epidemic of crippling workplace injuries.

These injuries, devastating as they are to a growing work force of committed caregivers, also point to a broader and equally dangerous problem. That problem is a developing crisis in staffing and conditions in nursing homes nationwide that threatens the quality of care for millions of America's most vulnerable citizens. It is a crisis that is occurring just as the $85 billion, mostly taxpayer-financed industry is experiencing its most radical transformation in a quarter century.

Occupational illness and injury rates for nursing home workers are higher than for workers in other industries with well-documented hazards, such as mining and construction.

More than 18 percent of all nursing home workers are injured or become ill on the job each year—more than twice the rate of private sector workers generally.

Occupational illness and injury rates for nursing home workers increased by 57 percent between 1984 and 1995, with more than 200,000 injuries reported in the industry every year.

Of those injured nursing home workers who must take time off, over a quarter require more than two work weeks to recover. Less than a third are able to return within one or two days.

Of the 20 fastest-growing industries in the United States, nursing homes have the highest rate of occupational illness and injury.

Back injuries, widely agreed to be among the most serious and costly of workplace injuries, are the most common type of injury suffered by nursing home workers.

While back injuries account for 27 percent of all injuries reported in the private sector, they account for 42 percent of all injuries in nursing homes.

Nurse aides, who provide most of the care in nursing homes, are particularly at risk.

Injuries to the back and trunk account for more than half of all injuries to nurse aides working in nursing homes.

The shift to prospective payment in both private and public health insurance has led to earlier hospital discharges and an overall increase in the acuity levels—the "sickness levels"—of nursing home patients. Unfortunately, staffing levels have not increased to match the increased workload.

Data from the federal On-Line Survey Certification and Reporting System (OSCARS) shows that the number of nurse aide hours per resident day only increased from 2.0 in 1992 to 2.1 in 1995, an insignificant amount.

Understaffing, according to a 1996 National Academy of Sciences' Institute of Medicine (IOM) report, leads to injuries, which leads to further understaffing. Nurse aides are often forced to lift residents alone when assistance is not immediately available. With sicker and more dependent residents, nursing homes have become more hazardous in terms of injuries.

The IOM report also states that research has demonstrated "a positive relationship between nursing staff levels and the quality of nursing home care, indicating a strong need to increase the overall level of nursing staff in nursing homes. [12]

Despite the obvious need for improvement, the funds provided do not allow managers of nursing homes to pay high wages. Nurses' aides – usually women performing difficult, thankless tasks, without much training – are paid extraordinarily low wages, while nurses fare little better. By the mid-1990s the salaries received by registered nurses in America were falling behind inflation. Wages rose only 3% from 1990 to 1994, and decreased by 1.5% between 1994 and 1997. [13]

Burnout rates are high, with staff changing frequently in any given nursing home, and under these circumstances, negligence and even patient abuse sometimes take place. Ironically, it may well be that

---

[12] Statistics and data referring here to the San Francisco Bay Area have been obtained from the following detailed study: Nursing Home Conditions in the San Francisco Bay Area: Many Homes Fail to Meet Federal Standards for Adequate Care, Minority Staff Special Investigations Division Committee on Government Reform U.S. House of Representatives, June 8, 2000.

[13] *The Shortage of Care*, a study by the SEIU Nursing Alliance.

the taxpayer is shelling out as much now to support the overworked healthcare professionals as would be necessary to simply hire more. Why? Because of the extremely high rate of injury and illness among nursing home employees, these are often in need of sick leave, of compensation and of other payments that could easily be avoided if staffing levels were reasonably high. In 1999, the occupational grouping of "RNs, nursing aides, and orderlies" reported work-related illnesses and injuries leading to 101,400 lost workdays. Registered nurses alone suffered 25,700 such illness and injuries in the same year. [14]

But what do the nurses themselves have to say about the crisis in healthcare today? The National Association of Geriatric Nursing Assistants testified before the US Senate Special Committee on aging in November 1999, with Debbie Byrd, certified nurses' aide as their representative. She presented a five point working plan that, if implemented, would only begin to address the issue. The five points were as follows:

1. Launch a national nursing assistant recruiting campaign.
2. Enact a government funded minimum wage for certified nurses' aides.
3. Avoid mandating minimum staffing ratios for nursing homes.
4. Establish a national registry of certified nurses' aides.
5. Support uniform national credential and education for certified nurses' aides.

These policies are simple and straightforward. Their implementation would represent a major advance, but would still fall short of correcting the problems in healthcare today. Medicare is more interested in reducing payments and reimbursements through audits, civil and criminal action and denial of claims than it is in the welfare of its beneficiaries. The government will not fund adequate wages for nurses' aides. The national average they receive is $7 an hour, ranging from as low as $5.45 an hour in rural areas to $12 an hour in urban areas. The modest goal of the NAGNA is to see wages increase to $10-12 an hour within the next two years. This is, quite simply, not going to happen. Ironically, the current situation of chronic understaffing was born when medical policies re-

---

[14] *The Shortage of Care*, a study by the SEIU Nursing Alliance.

duced the numbers of nurses in an attempt to cut costs. As the workforce declined in numbers, nursing became increasingly stressful, to the point where nurses left the profession for other jobs, and school leavers simply sought more attractive employment.

Sadly, many nurses are afraid of speaking aloud about the issue of understaffing. They fear retaliation or the loss of their jobs. Although little by little, the voices of nurses are added to the outcry against low staffing levels, public condemnation of this issue remains minimal.

So long as nursing homes are run as profit-generating businesses, and the government continues to establish regulations and rules demanding certain standards, nursing homes will be forced to choose only those residents that they can care for within their means. We will see more and more chain-operated nursing homes; "care franchises" if you will, where the individual needs of the patient are not respected, and the staff are not paid enough to stay and acquire the experience that makes them truly valuable.

Case Study: Portrait of a Nurses' Aide

Statistically speaking, most nurses' aides fall into a number of specific categories. Most are women, most are members of ethnic minorities, and few have a college education. Statistics, however, don't reveal anything about the people –the reasons behind their choice of career, their feelings about their work, and their reasons for going on. Meet Stephanie Cummins, certified nurses' aide.

"I decided to become a nurses' aide when I became interested in a career in nursing. My feeling was that starting here would be a positive step towards becoming a nurse, allowing me to learn about the profession from hands-on experience. I was also motivated by my interest in human behavior, and the opportunity to help sick, disabled and otherwise less privileged people. Taking care of others has always been a priority for me! At the risk of sounding vain, I feel that I can make a real difference in the lives of the elderly people I care for. I feel a lot of genuine love and compassion for them. Most of my colleagues have similar reasons for wanting to become certified nurses' aides, although we're all different – one went into the profession because she lacked the money to enter nursing college and I know of several who have families to support and would be prepared to do almost anything to keep going. Our ages are quite varied too. I work with a team of four, me and three other women, and our ages range from the early 20s to the early 60s. For some, being a nurses' aide is a first step towards a career in caregiving. For others, it can be a second or even third career. I'm 35 years old. I had my children early, and now that they're more independent, it's time I had a life of my own. I'm still young enough to train for a career, and I'm excited about the future!

Every day working in a nursing homes brings new challenges and difficulties, but there is one thing that never changes – we're always busy! Back pain and other problems are quite common among us all, as residents often have to be lifted, and the strain accumulates. The younger nurses' aides are more inclined to take risks, such as lifting people by themselves, but after a few years you start to learn how to be more careful. I won't say that every day brings great rewards, but there are times when you see how grateful the residents are for all you do for them, and that is wonderful. I have developed a relationship with some of the people I care for, but I can't help feeling that if staffing levels were even slightly higher, these relationships would be able to grow into real friendships. Some of the elderly people who live in the facility were I work crave affection, and it hurts not to be able to give them everything they need.

Case Study: Portrait of a Registered Nurse

Nurses are often described as "ministering angels". Carers they are, but angels they are not! Nurses are professionals. They want to help the sick and needy, but they also have very real concerns – family, financial obligations and more. Colette Colfer, 45, is a registered nurse. Until five years ago, she worked on the emergency ward of a large city hospital. When she and her family moved to the suburbs, she started to work in the local nursing home. Fortunately, her place of work is one of the better run establishments in her city, and she enjoys a good relationship with residents, other nurses and her superiors. Nonetheless, she is not surprised that her daughter is less than interested in the nursing profession. In a recent survey, [15] 32% of general, medical and surgical registered nurses said that they were unhappy with their current job situation,

---

[15] Reported in *Nursing Workforce Emerging Nurse Shortages due to Multiple Factors*, Report to the Chairman, Subcommittee on Health, Ways and Means, House of Representatives, United States General Accounting Office, July 2001.

while a survey of the American Nurses' Association revealed that a high percentage of nurses would not recommend their profession as a career choice to their own or others' children.

"I went to nursing school straight from high school and, apart from a few months maternity leave each time one of my three children was born, I have been working ever since. I'm lucky, in that I knew what I wanted to do, professionally, from an early age, and have been able to do so. Academically, I was quite a high achiever at high school and college. My ambitions, however, were not to become wealthy or famous, but to be able to spend my life helping others. A big inspiration was the fact that my younger sister was born with Turner's syndrome, and has lived with pain all her life. I've seen what a big difference quality nursing makes to the standard of living of the chronically ill.

I've spent most of my professional life working in emergency, so I've seen humanity at its worst, and at its best. I've dealt with drug addicts overdosing, accident victims, coronary victims, gang members wounded in shoot-outs ... everything. I was always able to take it in my stride, and I've often been impressed with the ability of people –mothers, husbands, wives – to deal with trauma.

I started working in the nursing home industry five years ago. The biggest difference between working here and working in emergency is that on an emergency ward, the fight is to keep people alive. Many of the patients are young, and if the medical staff can stop them from dying, have their best years ahead of them. In a nursing home, it's different. Most of the residents are old, and while we place an emphasis on the home as a place to live, it's also a place to try and die with dignity. When you are ninety years old, the best part of your life is behind you.

To some people, it seems depressing to work with the old and the dying. To a nurse, it's not. To me, a peaceful, dignified death is less frightening than a tortured life. The home where I work is one of the best in the state. Medicare beneficiaries and other residents are all treated equally, and administration does its best to care for the elderly patients as well as possible. We have the usual problems of underfunding and understaffing, but strive to do our best despite the frustrations, such as not being able to spend as much time with each patient as he or she deserves. The fact that this is a small, privately run home helps. With no more than 60 residents at any one time, even the administrators know the patients by name.

Of course, things are not ideal. At the moment, each nurses' aide is responsible for eight residents. This means that they simply don't have enough time to feed everyone with the proper amount of patience and care. At any one time, at least two or three of the nursing staff is suffering from backache or headache from the stress of trying to fit everything in. I know that we are all worried about the future, too. The nursing population is aging. What will happen when we are in our late fifties and early sixties? That's too young to retire, but by then it may be more difficult to lift and bathe people.

My daughter, Ethel, is fifteen years old, and thinking about what she wants to do when she finishes high school. When I suggested nursing to her, she looked at me as if I had gone mad.

"No way," she said, "I'm not going to work as hard as you do for that kind of money." She has a point. She wants to live in the city, be independent. My husband is an accountant, and earns more than twice as much as me, enabling us to run a comfortable home. But what if Ethel doesn't marry someone with a higher earning capacity? Or doesn't marry at all? She has the right to a decent standard of living. The last time we talked about her career options, she said that she was thinking of going into computer programming.

Discrepancies in Care

The quality of care given in many homes is demonstrably less than ideal. A huge percentage fail to pass the health and safely standards – many patients are found to be suffering from conditions that are avoidable, such as bedsores, unnecessary pain and other symptoms that seriously compromise their quality of life and sense of dignity. Many patients experience a rapid decline in physical and psychological health on entering a nursing home, and depression is common – hardly surprising, as caregivers change frequently and have little time to talk, making it difficult to form the sort of emotional, compassionate relationship necessary to maintain psychological health. The issue of understaffing underpins every deficit in nursing homes today, and this is a constant theme of this book.

The quality of life and standard of care available varies widely from one home to the next, even among those institutions that are shown to comply with identical federal healthcare regulations. But how can such discrepancies exist? Perhaps we should look at how good nursing homes are run. They have a higher ratio of nurses to residents, a low turnover of employees and key employees who may have been employed for years. Staff members are compassionate and committed to caring for the elderly. But even America's very best nursing homes are inadequate. They lack the resources to remodel, conduct research and recruit and hire highly educated professionals who will contribute to the bettering of nursing home care, and long-term care in general. All nursing homes are caught in a sort of time warp, providing the same service year after year after year. We expect supermarkets and car manufacturers to adapt their products as time passes – we should demand no less of nursing homes and cease to accept care standards that have remained unchanged for three decades. Would you like to shop for your weekly groceries in a supermarket of the 1950s? Probably not. And neither should you accept that our nursing homes offer the same type and standard of care available a generation ago.

State Monitoring of Healthcare Facilities

The Department of Health and Human Services usually contracts with the various state Departments of Health to provide certification and annual inspections of nursing homes. Inspectors are told to look for indications that predefined standards of care are being met, including the prevention of bedsores, general hygiene conditions and the prevention of accidents. While many homes fail to reach acceptable levels, some err more seriously than others. To describe the degree of negligence, four general categories of violation of the health laws have been devised: those which may lead to slight harm to a resident; those which might lead to more serious harm; those that cause actual harm and – and it is a shame that the following category exists at all – those that cause actual death or have the potential to cause actual death or serious injury. Inspections at national and state level have revealed many inadequate nursing homes, but inspectors are quick to point out that shortcomings in healthcare facilities can be addressed relatively quickly, by increasing staffing levels, replacing business-minded directors with directors who care, and by ensuring that there are adequate funds to meet patients' needs.

A recent study conducted in the San Francisco Bay Area of California [16], revealed deeply worrying trends. Only 18 homes in the area were found to be in full or substantial compliance with federal standards in 2000, while 119 (more than one-third, catering to more than 13,000 residents) were found to have violations that caused serious harm to their residents – even placing them at risk of injury or death. Deficiencies included the failure to prevent or properly treat pressure sores, preventable accidents, inadequate medical treatment, and the failure to provide proper nutrition or hydration. The homes with actual harm violations were estimated in 2000 to receive $141 million each year in federal and state funds.

Lamentably, the methods of enforcing changes are a part of the problem, and not the solution. Inspection agencies are enforcers. Their role is to approve statistics submitted by homes in order to prove that the job of care-taking is being done properly. Inspectors do not correct, change or offer advice to improve the quality of care in nursing homes, resembling more closely the highway patrol than representatives of an institution designed to enhance the quality of life. Just as the issuing of fines for speeding does not reduce the level of traffic violations, the issuing of fines to nursing homes does not reduce the rate of elder abuse and neglect. In each case, the purse of government is swollen.

Homes Run as Businesses

Without complete government subsidization for nursing homes, they are inevitably run as businesses, and as with every business, attempts must be made to make the overheads as low as possible – to maximize profit. Throughout the 1990s, nursing homes became increasingly consolidated, until the five largest chains operated over 2,000 facilities, buying up small and privately owned homes. Huge numbers of residents, and large sums of money are involved in these nursing home giants. When something goes wrong, large chains have the means to pay for the best legal representation there is. Authorities are reluctant to target such superpowers and, instead, have opted for making examples of small homes, leading to bank-

---

[16] Report to Congress 2000, *Appropriateness of Minimum Nurse Staffing Ratios in Nursing homes.*

ruptcy and increased consolidation. Of course, there are many fine healthcare workers employed by chains – but there are also many managers whose bottom line is the almighty dollar, and not the quality of life of their residents. Thus, some nursing home managers require their nurses' aides to work as quickly as they can, in getting their elderly patients in and out of bed, in feeding them, changing their clothes and helping them to attend to their hygiene needs. Working at speed does not leave much time for the type of attention that makes life worth living – forming personal relationships and constructing friendships – let alone attending to sick, old people's bodily requirements. The importance of emotional ties between staff and residents is evinced by more than just anecdotal evidence; in a report to Congress in year 2000 [17] this crucial aspect of quality care was underlined.

... patients and nursing staff regard the relationship that develops between a vulnerable adult and her caregiver to be of paramount importance in determining the quality of a resident's life. Residents describe the importance of gentleness, personal engagement, not being rushed and feeling respected. Aides report that they value having time to promote physical comfort, not make residents wait or rush, and share treats or personal stories ... over time .. residents gradually become more accepting of care if well-trained and supervised staff members are available to permit development of personal rapport.

In the long-term, greater staffing levels and more intensive nursing care reduce costs. Patients who are allowed to visit the toilet frequently have less need of incontinence pads. Patients who are helped to move around and exercise are less likely to develop bedsores or other problems associated with immobility. Patients who develop warm relationships with caring staff members are less likely to become depressed. The more comfortable the patient is, and the happier, the less likely he or she is to develop a wide range of problems, ultimately leading to reduced medical spending. None of this can occur, however, without substantial public investment *no*w. The homes that currently provide the worst care are those run by large profit-driven corporations, and especially chains. These are administered in a way not much different to any MacDonald's

---

[17] Report to Congress 2000, *Appropriateness of Minimum Nurse Staffing Ratios in Nursing homes*.

outlet, with patients' considerations coming well below profit margins in terms of importance to the investors.

What is a Typical Day in a Run-as-a-Business Nursing Home Really Like?

Let's take a look at a typical day in one of those homes where the care of the residents comes in way behind profit margins in terms of priority. Although there are plenty of real homes that I could pinpoint, for legal reasons this is a fictionalized account of knowledge I have of a number of such establishments. Any similarities of names of either people or facility to real persons or places are coincidental.

7:30 – 8.00 a.m.

The residents' day at Peach Valley nursing home begins when the sleepy nurses' aides start to wheel around the breakfast trolleys. Toast and breakfast cereals are what are usually on the menu, although some of the residents find it hard to manage the crunchy flakes. About half of the 250 patients are unable to eat alone, and need to be spoon-fed – but each nurses' aide is responsible for feeding at least ten old people, and breakfast has to be finished by 8:15 at the latest. Inevitably, many residents can't finish their food, which is cleared away before they've satisfied their appetites. Today, Annie Green choked on a spoonful of milk-soaked cereal. She doesn't usually have any trouble eating, but the nurses' aide, rushing to finish feeding her and move on to the next patient, spooned the soggy mixture into her mouth too quickly. Now Annie's throat hurts, and she will have to be fed liquids until it's better. Patty, the responsible nurses' aide, feels horribly guilty. She is fond of Annie, and meant no harm, but felt herself under pressure to finish breakfast and get on to the next task of the day.

8.00 a.m. – 12.00 p.m.

While the nurses' aides hurry residents through their baths, change their diapers and bedclothes and listen to their complaints and worries, the registered nurses make the rounds of the rooms with medication for the patients. Residents with diabetes need to have their insulin levels checked, those on ventilators need to have the machines tubes changed. Those with Alzheimer's disease are kept under restraints, some by being physically tied into their beds or wheelchairs, and others by being kept under heavy sedation. This is far from being the ideal way of caring for confused elders, but staffing levels are not high enough to ensure that they will not wander off, become aggressive, or do themselves some harm in another way. A few of the residents are well enough to get out of bed, and they shuffle, in varying states of undress, to the activity room where John and Sandy, young volunteers from the community, have arranged some simple activities such as card games and artwork, to keep their minds as active as possible. John and Sandy do their best to help in their free time, but they are not professional therapists, and are not able to cope with all the residents' needs. Paula Smith, a resident who, at ninety, is only slightly confused, loves to play cards. She is incontinent, however, and the nurses' aides have forgotten to make sure that her diaper has been changed. Remarks from other residents about the smell reduce her to tears.

At eleven, the director of the nursing home, Mary Bryan, calls a staff meeting, leaving a handful of nurses' aides to oversee the residents. Ms. Bryan is a graduate of the Chicago School of Business. Before she went into nursing home management, she ran a small chain of hardware stores. Financially speaking, the change of business has been good for her – her income has more than doubled in the last five years. At the meeting she announces further cutbacks. The facility has been spending too much money on certain items, including the latex gloves worn by nurses and nurses' aides to prevent the spread of infection from one resident to the next. From now on, the supply of latex gloves will be kept to a strict minimum. After the meeting, she draws Leroy Jones, the only male nurses' aide, aside and tells him that his services are no longer needed. The facility can't afford to pay for him any more. He will be sorely missed by his colleagues, who had come to rely on him to control distressed male patients, and to lift the heavier residents in and out of the bath.

At eleven-thirty the nursing director, Margaret Chan, is taken aback when a resident's daughter storms into her office to complain.

"My father has lost over twenty-five pounds in the last fortnight," she says, close to tears, "I'd take him out if only there were somewhere else for him to go".

Margaret soothes her and promises to review her father's diet chart, but she knows that the basic problem is simply that the nurses' aides can't afford to spend half an hour with each patient making sure they eat.

The Crisis in America's Nursing Homes

12.00 p.m.- 1.00 p.m.

It's lunch time, and although many of the morning's chores are left undone, the nurses' aides have to stop what they are doing to bring around the food – chicken soup followed by a stew with vegetables and prawns. Esther Goldstein, one of the facilities residents, is Jewish and cannot eat shellfish because she is committed to a kosher diet. Today, she will go without lunch. Nobody notices that she has not eaten, and her attempts to get the attention of her nurses' aide go unacknowledged.

1:00 p.m.- 5.00 p.m.

Today, the facility's doctor makes his monthly visit. If a resident needs to see a doctor during the rest of the month, he or she is taken to the emergency ward in the hospital. Doing the rounds, he finds four residents with new bedsores, and also discovers one old man with a bed sore that has deteriorated so much from last month, that his hip bone has become visible. He increases the dose of antibiotics to each of these residents and stresses once more the importance of turning old people regularly to prevent pressure sores from appearing in the first place. On his way out the door, he is accosted by one of the residents with Alzheimer's disease, ninety-two year old Lawrence Moss. Lawrence had been tied into his bed but has managed to work his bonds loose.

"Take me out of here, Johnny," Lawrence cries as he clutches the doctor's sleeve. Johnny was Lawrence's son, who died in Vietnam thirty years ago. Two nurses' aides come forward to take the sobbing Lawrence back to his room and give him a sedative.

At three in the afternoon, the evening shift staff clock in, and the morning staff is free to go home. There is no overlap of time, as the directorship is reluctant to pay a cent more than necessary, so the morning's nurses' aides don't have time to tell their colleagues who has been changed today and who has not, who is feeling gloomy and who is reasonably content.

5.00 p.m. -7.00 p.m.

Before the evening meal is served, the local Catholic and Episcopalian pastors make their rounds, dispensing communion and comfort to those residents that are members of their respective churches. Father Brian expresses concern about the unpleasant smell in the nursing facility – the result of too many unchanged diapers and unwashed sheets – but he is paid little attention and is reluctant to hassle the obviously stressed nurses and nurses' aides.

7.00 p.m. - 8.00 p.m.

Time for the evening meal of macaroni and cheese. Because it's easy to eat, this is a favorite of many residents and even Mrs. Goldstein manages to get some of it down. Once the meal is over, it is time to start getting residents into bed and ready for the night shift. All of the residents, including those with no problems of incontinence, are fitted with two sets of diapers, because there isn't enough night staff to help people visit the bathroom.

9.00 p.m.

City Hall is holding a reception for local businesses, and Mary Bryan, as the director of one of the more flourishing ventures, has been invited to attend. She has prepared a speech for the occasion: "Making business work in the New Millennium."

Mary Bryan spends a lot of money on health insurance. She has no intention of ever ending up in a nursing facility like the one she runs.

What is a Typical Day in a Nursing Home with Proper, Professional Staffing Really Like?

Nursing homes don't have to be as bleak as the one in the picture we painted above. There are some homes where the residents live out the rest of their lives in dignity, where relatives can visit and leave knowing that their parents or loved ones are well-cared for and happy.

7:00 a.m.

The day shift nurses, still a bit sleepy, report on duty. Before they leave, those who worked the previous shift give them a report of how the night went – Mrs. Giusti in room 3 slept badly, they'll need to be particularly gentle with her, Tom Jones in room 5 has a slight cold, and needs to be watched. Before reaching the residents' rooms, the staff as a whole discusses the events of the day. The nurses in charge discuss the physicians' appointments, and individual residents needs are discussed in detail with the certified nurses' aides. In Lakeview nursing home, each charge nurse oversees a team of four certified nurses' aides, and each nurses' aide is assigned the care of four residents for her shift. Residents' progress is also monitored and supervised by charge nurses, who are responsible for 16 patients each.

The certified nurses' aides who work in Lakeside are the envy of their colleagues in other, less well run nursing homes. Here, management recognizes that they are crucial to ensure that the residents are well cared-for, and that all their needs are being met. It is never forgotten that a resident's needs are not just physical. Their emotional requirements are just as important, as is retaining as much autonomy over their lives as possible. With only four residents to care for, each nurses' aide has time to provide all the support they need.

8:00 a.m. – 11:00 a.m.

After the charge nurses have discussed the activities of the day and the medical and emotional status of the patients with the aides, breakfast is served to the patients. It's a beautiful day, so the morning meal is served outside, on the patio. The residents always enjoy the opportunity to feel the sunshine on their faces. On duty since 7 a.m. Anna, one of Lakeside's most well-liked nurses' aides, has had time to make sure that her four charges are up and dressed in time to eat. When the kitchen staff arrive with the food, Anna helps to serve it, and she also sits and talks with the group about the events that have been planned for the day: therapy schedules, care conferences and activities. She runs through the meal plan for tomorrow to make sure that there are no objections to the menu. A chorus of groans greets the news that spinach is planned as the vegetable dish, so Anna notes that an alternative should be provided for those who are not fond of it. Some exciting trips have been planned for later in the week, including a visit to the mall, and a nature walk.

The charge nurse drops by the patio area, too, to deliver medication to residents, and to discuss and coordinate events and activities with teams, just so as to ensure that plans are not in conflict. One big issue is taking care that no space is double-booked. Space is always a problem. So many activities are on offer, that the staff members have to be careful that there's a place for everybody. In fact, later today the management has agreed to meet to look into ways to increase living space. Today, the charge nurses are meeting with family members to discuss the progress and condition of residents. At Lakeview, a monthly patient care conference is held, together with both resident and family to discuss the residents' needs, desires and treatment plan.

Anna has been working here for five years, and has been caring for the same residents for many months. As she clears away the breakfast things, she chats with the residents, who know her by name and ask with interest how her children are getting along in school. With all sincerity, Anna feels that she can consider the residents to be friends and not just responsibilities. Without having to rush through her work, she has had time to discuss their interests and hobbies. Of course, the faces change, as residents leave the home, or as their lives draw to a close. But each new group becomes almost like a family.

"It's like the family I grew up in," Anna thinks. She has two brothers and a sister. They drove each other crazy at times when they were kids, but they always looked out for each other, swapped news at the end of the day and each felt part of a team. "Her" residents have also grown close, and even their families get together to talk and exchange news when they meet in the home. How different it is in Lakeside than in the previous nursing home in which Anna worked! There, she had to take care of seven or eight residents, often different people every day. She never even had time to learn their names. Although she had gone into the caring profession because she wanted to make a difference, her job quickly became routine, rushing through the paces so as to finish everything as quickly as possible.

11:00 a.m. – 1:00 p.m.

Anna noticed over breakfast that Mr. Jones was not his usual, cheerful self, so she spends some extra time with him before lunch. Of course, she has to look after the other residents, too, but fortunately she's not under pressure to finish everything quickly, and so she has some time to sit and wait. He's running a slight fever because he has a cold, and is feeling depressed. Although his wife died eight years ago, he still misses her every day. "I'm useless without her," he mutters miserably, "I'm just a useless old man waiting to die." Anna gradually introduces other topics into the conversation, by pointing to the photographs of his grandchildren on the bedside locker and asking how they are getting on at school. Pretty soon the proud grandfather is boasting about how little Emmett scored a try last week. He's almost forgotten about his cold and is thinking about the future instead of dwelling on the past. Lunch is served at one, and Anna has to help the kitchen staff with the dishes and assist two of her residents with their meals, but by this time, Mr. Jones is as upbeat as ever.

The Crisis in America's Nursing Homes

2:00 p.m. – 4:00 p.m.

After lunch, a group of the more mobile residents is taken on a shopping trip. It's October, and Lakeview nursing home encourages the local children to drop by when they go trick or treating. With the help of their attendants, the residents shop for candy and other treats, almost as excited as the kids will be later on. At the home, another small group sees their physical therapist, Gemma. It's important for them to exercise their muscles often. Inactivity can lead to deterioration of muscle tone to the extent that the patient can become bedridden and this, in turn, can lead to the risk of pressure sores and other ailments associated with old age. Gemma manages to make the exercise fun, and at the end of the session the residents are tired, but laughing. During this time, the registered nurses write their reports of the shift, and the nurses' aides attend to their duties and take note of any special issues that should be reported to the evening shift. The staff for the evening shift clocks in at 3.30, leaving time for communication between the two groups of workers. Before she leaves for home, Anna tells her replacement, a young woman who has only been working at Lakeside for a fortnight, that Mr. Jones has been a bit depressed, and has a cold. Sue, the new aide, promises to keep an eye on him.

5:00 p.m. – 9:00 p.m.

It's been a busy day for the residents at Lakeside! Most of them are tired, and the evening is spent quietly, with some napping, some reading newspapers or magazines, and some chatting with visitors. Nurses' aides are never far from their assigned residents. At six, a light evening meal is served, and by nine, most residents are ready for bed, although a few opt to stay up to watch television. The director of Lakeside, John Cohen, who was at a symposium about the use of massage care of the elderly, drops by in the evening to talk to the nurses in charge and make sure that everything ran smoothly in his absence. On hearing that there were no problems, he bids the staff good night and leaves for home. He'll be back at work tomorrow morning at nine.

Like so many problems, the nursing home crisis boils down to a relatively small number of key points, some practical, and others stemming from generalized attitudes towards nursing care. Abundantly clear is the fact that the nursing profession does not receive the respect it deserves, and that nursing is a profoundly undervalued profession in modern America. The reasons for the customary undervaluing of nursing are manifold – some point to the fact that it has, in a patriarchal society, traditionally been dominated by women, others to low rates of unionization and others to the fact that it tends to be seen as a "vocation" rather than a job, like a calling to ministry, or taking vows in a convent. The truth incorporates all of this, and more. A common perception of the nurse is that she or he is there to soothe and comfort patients, rather than take responsibility for their lives and the ease of their deaths. Although medical doctors could not function without nurses, who deal with the intimate realities of illness and disability on a daily basis, they are seen very much as second rate personnel in healthcare, and are paid accordingly.

Understaffing [18]

If there is one thing that social researchers, concerned healthcare workers, nursing home residents and the families of residents agree upon, it is that staffing levels in America's nursing homes are far too low. Recommended staffing levels are as follows: a "preferred minimum" level whereby each resident receives 3.45 hours of nursing care per day, of which two are provided by nursing assistants, one by a registered or licensed nurse, and the rest by a registered nurse. The few homes that correspond to this level of staffing provide a demonstrably higher service to their patients. A lower minimum level of staffing has also been identified, with 2.95 hours of nursing care per resident per day, with less time given to licensed and registered nurses. A majority of nursing facilities fails to reach even the lower of the two designated standards, while even those facilities that would like to increase their staffing levels to reasonable levels have difficulty doing so, as the nursing profession fails to attract new recruits, and loses qualified nurses to work-related ailments or simple burn-out.

---

[18] Two sources in particular have been useful in obtaining the statistics quoted here; *Nursing Workforce Emerging Nurse Shortages due to Multiple Factors*, Report to the Chairman, Subcommittee on Health, Ways and Means, House of Representatives, United States General Accounting Office, July 2001, and *The Shortage of Care*, a study by the SEIU Nursing Alliance.

When the Nursing Facility Staffing Improvement Act was passed in 2000, State Inspectors were given more authority to penalize facilities for inadequate staffing levels, allowing them to examine the role that understaffing plays in patient neglect and abuse, pinpointing the offending homes, and ensuring that they take steps to redress the problem.

There is a direct correlation between the numbers of nursing staff and the quality of life – and life expectancy – of the residents. Lower numbers of staff mean that elderly patients cannot always be taken to attend to their physical functions, and devices such as catheters may be used for patients for whom they should not be necessary. Lower staffing rates invariably lead to a higher incidence of skin infection, urinary tract infection, sores, poor physical function, and emotional stress. Malnutrition, dehydration and other avoidable conditions occur – not because the nursing staff is necessarily negligent or under qualified, but because they are simply too few in number to devote enough time to each individual patient. A recently published academic paper about standards in nursing homes reported the following scenario.

> ... because the food carts had to be returned to the kitchen at a specific time, the staff had only 45 minutes to an hour to feed residents. Feeling pressured to finish within the hour, the staff became impatient with those who ate slowly. They talked to them authoritatively: "Open your mouth!" "Don't talk, eat!" "Laura, keep quiet. Laura, be quiet, you're eating." ... When residents ate too slowly, the staff often mixed the solid food ... with the liquids ... the entree, the vegetables and the dessert were added to the milk, resulting in an unidentifiable, unpalatable mixture. Sometimes residents were forced to eat rapidly against their wishes; huge spoonfuls of food were placed in their mouths. Some residents coughed and choked as they were fed too quickly. [19]

Managers with their eye on their profit margins go for short-term gain, cutting corners in staff recruitment, reducing the standard of living of their residents and, ultimately, making healthcare even more expensive as avoidable health problems are not prevented.

---

[19] Kayser-Jones and Schell, "The effect of staffing on the quality of care at mealtime", Nursing Outline, 1997, 45.

Let me stress once more. Understaffing is *serious*. It leads to sickness – both of residents and of overworked nurses and nurses' aides – and even to death. In the San Francisco Bay Area study, researchers revealed an alarming situation. In one case, a facility's failure to care for a resident's sores led to the amputation of her left leg. In another, a resident's feeding tube was not monitored, and the patient died of the cardiopulmonary arrest and pneumonia that resulted from overfeeding. A diabetic patient was not provided with insulin, and as a result his leg was amputated. A patient was found with ants crawling in and out of her mouth, and another with a larvae infested wound. The depressing list goes on and on. In homes containing seriously confused or senile patients, staff members have not always been present in sufficient numbers to prevent violent or confrontational residents from attacking others and doing them physical harm. Extremely common, due to low staffing levels, is a failure to ensure that residents are not forced to sit in their own urine and feces. [20] Residents and nursing staff members are not merely statistics. They are citizens, and they are entitled to a better healthcare system.

Inadequate staffing levels also have a negative effect on the physical and emotional health of nursing staff, who become vulnerable to repetitive stress injury and psychological pressure that can lead to a complete emotional breakdown. Again, the long-term costs of recruiting nursing staff members are higher as individual workers are obliged, for health reasons, to take time off work or leave the profession completely.

Already, there is insufficient qualified nursing staff to run the nation's nursing homes. This problem will grow in the years to

---

[20] Statistics and data referring here to the San Francisco Bay Area have been obtained from the following detailed study: *Nursing Home Conditions in the San Francisco Bay Area: Many Homes Fail to Meet Federal Standards for Adequate Care*, Minority Staff Special Investigations Division Committee on Government Reform U.S. House of Representatives, June 8, 2000.

come [21] The nursing population, like the general population, is getting older, with the average age of nurses significantly higher than it was twenty or even ten years ago. Replacement levels are low, with nursing no longer a popular career option among young women, who traditionally formed the majority of the profession. Reasons for a decline of interest in nursing are not hard to identify. Remuneration is low, working conditions are often poor, nurses are among the most at risk for work related injury or illness, and the profession as whole is not greatly respected. At the time of writing, nurses can reasonably expect to reach their maximum earning capacity within five to seven years of entering the profession, creating an environment in which there is little initiative to strive for improvement. The hourly rate charged by non-medical professionals and tradesman exceeds by far that paid to nurses. Attorneys can earn from $100 to $500 per hour, auto mechanics from $35 to $85 per hour, but nurses, who are responsible for the welfare of our elderly parents and grandparents, earn a fraction of these sums. If earning capacity is any indication of the esteem in which the government and the tax paying public holds its healthcare professionals, these are surely an undervalued group in society! Why, in these circumstances, would bright young high school graduates even consider nursing as a valid career option? It is important to recognize nurses as the highly qualified healthcare professionals that they are, and attempts will have to be made to attract intelligent, capable and dedicated young people of *bot*h sexes into the profession. A recent study describes the situation more than clearly:

Current problems with the recruitment and retention of nurses are related to multiple factors. The nurse workforce is aging, and fewer new nurses are entering the profession to replace those who are retiring or leaving. Furthermore, nurses report unhappiness with many aspects of the work environment including staffing levels, heavy workloads, increased use of overtime, lack of sufficient support staff, and inadequate wages. In many cases this growing dissatisfaction is affecting their decisions to remain in nursing. The decline in younger people, predominantly women, choosing nursing as a career has re-

---

[21] Figures quoted here come from: *Staffing of Nursing Services in Long-term Care: Present Issues and Prospects for the future* prepared by, Health Services Research and Evaluation, American Healthcare Association.

sulted in a steadily aging RN workforce. Over the last two decades, as opportunities for women outside of nursing have expanded, the number of young women entering the RN workforce has declined [22]

All of the projections suggest that the nursing workforce will continue to age. [23] Since 1983, the average age of working registered nurses has increased from 37.4 to 45.2. To date, the average age of the workforce of registered nurses is increasing *twice as quickly* as that of the workforce as a whole. By 2010, as much as 40% of the workplace will be over 50, and it has been predicted that by 2020 the nursing population will run at numbers 20% below those necessary to keep the facilities open, or at a deficit of around 400,000. In fact, female high school graduates were, throughout the 1990s, 35% less likely to enter nursing school than in the 1970s. As always, few men enter the profession, and this is unlikely to change as long as government and society undervalue the profession. Those nurses who entered the workforce in the 1970s are now in their 40s and will themselves be approaching retirement age when the tidal wave of baby boomers becomes elderly and in need of care. Again, I quote:

The large numbers of RNs that entered the labor force in the 1970s are now over the age of 40 and are not being replenished by younger RNs. Between 1983 and 1998, the number of RNs in the workforce under 30 fell by 41 percent, compared to only a 1 percent decline in the number under age 30 in the rest of the U.S. workforce.

Over the past 2 decades, the nurse workforce's average age has climbed steadily. While over half of all RNs were reported to be under age 40 in 1980, fewer than one in three were younger than 40 in 2000 ... the age distribution of RNs has shifted dramatically upward. The percent of nurses under age 30 decreased from 26 percent in 1980 to 9 percent in 2000, while the percentage 40 to 49 grew from 20 to 35 percent. In addition to the lack of students en-

---

[22] *Nursing Workforce Emerging Nurse Shortages due to Multiple Factors*, Report to the Chairman, Subcommittee on Health, Ways and Means, House of Representatives, United States General Accounting Office, July 2001.

[23] GAO analysis of US Census Bureau Projections of Total Resident Population, Middle Series, December 1999.

tering and graduating from nursing programs, there is concern about a pending shortage of nurse educators. The average age of professors in nursing programs is 52, and 49 for associate professors. [24]

Nurses are not happy, and they have good reason. Many are dissatisfied with the low salaries they receive, while others are concerned about the effect that understaffing in hospitals and nursing homes has on their health. They are not content with the level of recognition they get from their employers. The central role of nursing care facilities in American healthcare is increasing, as subacute facilities continue to become more important. Wages for the nurses that work in these facilities come mostly from Medicare and Medicaid funding, and as such they are calculated on the basis of historic wage levels, and not on the demands and necessities of current times. Nurses working in subacute care facilities or nursing homes earn substantially less that their colleagues in hospitals, who are somehow perceived to have more "glamorous" or "important" roles.

Nurses tend to move from one nursing facility to another in the search for adequate working conditions and pay, but understaffing is endemic, and for most this is a thankless quest.

Case Study: Portrait of a Student Nurse

The future of the healthcare system in the United States depends upon the healthcare workers of the future. However, many potential nurses and nurses' aides look at a system riddled with problems – underfunding, understaffing, low wages and low social esteem for its employees – and decide to seek their fortune elsewhere. Meet Debbie Coleman, from Ohio. Debbie is in her second year of nursing training.

Debbie was a bright, successful high school student whose final examination results would have been good enough for her to enroll in a university program. But she has known since she was only fourteen that she wanted to work in a

---

[24] *Nursing Workforce Emerging Nurse Shortages due to Multiple Factors*, Report to the Chairman, Subcommittee on Health, Ways and Means, House of Representatives, United States General Accounting Office, July 2001

caring profession. Her parents operate a veterinary practice so she is familiar with animal medicine, but Debbie is more interested in human patients.

The first year of training was tough, but interesting, and fuelled Debbie's commitment even further. During this year she met her boyfriend Paul, a student on the same course. Like Debbie, Paul is an intelligent young person who could just as easily have studied for a more lucrative career at the state university, but who feels that the healthcare industry will be more rewarding emotionally and intellectually than a job shuffling papers in an office. Debbie and Paul accept the fact that they will never be rich – although they do hope that there will be some reforms in nurses' pay before they graduate.

Now, half way through her second year of nursing school, Debbie is beginning to have serious reservations about the career she has chosen for herself. Her doubts do not spring from worries about her interest in the profession, but from her experience during the Summer vacation. While many classmates took temporary jobs in clothing stores or in fast food outlets, Debbie opted to work as a nurses' aide in one of the homes near her parents' house. Her fifteen year old brother, flipping burgers at a nearby drive-in for the Summer season, brought home a bigger wage package than she did, but Debbie felt that the experience would be valuable.

Before she began her Summer job, Debbie was sure that she was under no illusions as to how difficult it was going to be. She was prepared to have to lift heavy, incapacitated residents, to soothe the worries of confused elderly patients, and to work long hours for little compensation.

The reality of working in Oak Lawns nursing home was far worse that she could ever have imagined.

On her first day at work, Debbie was put in the charge of Tiffany, a thirty year old nurses' aide with several years' experience. The registered nurse in charge outlined their duties for the day, and the two set off to give breakfast to the residents. Debbie was shocked by the torrent of racist abuse hurled at Tiffany by a number of the residents, who suffer from Alzheimer's disease. Tiffany, who is originally from the Philippines, shrugged it off.

"You get used to it," she said, "Poor things. They have no idea where they are or who I am."

Throughout the summer months, Debbie grew to know several of the nurses' aides and registered nurses well. Tempers could be short in the nursing home – the hours they work are long, and the job is stressful – but, by and large, she was impressed by their dedication to their work. However, many of the things she witnessed in Oak Lawns horrified her. In July, one of the nurses had to take early retirement. The back injury she had sustained three years ago when she had to lift a wheelchair-bound patient by herself just became too much to cope with. She is only fifty years old – too young to retire, yet at an age when it's hard to start a second career. Later the same month, a new resident was admitted. Lynda Potter was suffering from severe malnutrition. A Medicare beneficiary, her payments did not cover the medications she needed for her angina and osteoporosis conditions, and she had been cutting back on food for months to pay for them. Lynda, who is in her eighties, is not remotely confused and should not be in a nursing home. If her payments had been sufficient, her condition would not have deteriorated to such an extent, and she would have been able to stay in her home. In August, Tiffany quit her job as nurses' aide, and went to work as a waitress in a seafood restaurant. With her pleasant personality and bright smile, she'll be able to make more in tips that she ever could earn in a nursing home.

Things are not as tough for registered nurses as they are for nurses' aides – but they are still far from ideal. When Debbie returned to college in the Fall, she was depressed and disillusioned. Her boyfriend Paul, who spend the Summer working in his parents' mechanic shop, tried to cheer her up, telling her that she doesn't have to work in a nursing home, that things will be better by the time they graduate, and that the system must be changed from within.

"The healthcare system needs people like you and me," he insists. Paul is right. The healthcare system does need dedicated, intelligent young professionals. But why should Debbie, who is now seriously thinking of leaving nursing college to train as a legal secretary, continue her studies to enter a profession where she will be underpaid, disrespected and even subjected to abuse when frustrated families lash out against a system that is neglecting their loved ones?

To attract young people into the nursing profession, money will have to be spent by the government and the taxpayer, and again, an initial investment will result in lower spending in the long-term. Adequate compensation for nursing professionals will lead to higher rates of recruitment from among the best high school graduates. A well-trained and educated nursing staff will take better care of the nation's sick and elderly citizens, who will then enjoy better rates of recovery and ultimately incur less cost to the taxpayer.

The situation in American's nursing homes is bleak and, despite the best efforts of some nursing home administrators, the prognosis for the future is not bright. Since 1998, at least one fifth of the nursing homes in Washington State have been forced to declare themselves bankrupt, and other states fare little better [25]

Prescription for a Better Future

To provide our senior citizens with the care they need, we need to set staffing levels at 6.2 hours per patient, per day. Any less, and we risk failing to secure optimum health levels and rewarding lives for the elders among us. To put it bluntly, if we fail to provide this standard of nursing, we are warehousing our senior citizens, and setting up a care system that is substandard.

Just to provide nursing home residents with the basics of care – meaningful personal contact, medication, treatments, water, food, clothing and hygiene – a facility should maintain minimum staffing levels of one nurses' assistant for every four residents for sixteen hours a day and one nurses' aide for every eight residents during the night. There should also be one licensed nurse assigned to each sixteen residents for the sixteen hours of the day and one registered nurse assigned to every thirty-two residents at night. A nursing home also needs a social worker, an activity leader, a director of nurses, an assistant director of nurses and a supervisor of nursing for infection control. Quality monitoring and additional support staff should be on hand to carry out regulatory functions. The facility should also employ a physical therapist, a speech therapist and an occupational therapist with their respective support staff. A department of education should be established for each facility. Please note that I am referring only to basic care. Residents with specialized medical needs require much, much more.

Ideally, nursing homes that currently house residents in shared bedrooms should convert these to single rooms so as to allow residents to bring items from home. Personal furniture and paintings, pictures of family and personal possessions all enhance the residents' quality of life and make nursing homes more pleasant

---

[25] Heath Foster, *Washington Post*, April 28, 2000.

places to live, visit and work in. It sounds simple, doesn't it? Yet none of this will happen in today's nursing home industry. There are three main reasons for this – the government, the industry and the public. The government and the public do not want to pay for the cost of additional staffing, education and space. The nursing home industry does not want more regulations or the complications attached to increased funding. Nursing homes are not seen as homes, but as a series of beds to be filled. Beds are either occupied or unoccupied, and every empty bed is seen merely as a potential for generating more money. Many nursing home managers concentrate on filling as many beds as possible rather than on ways to make the residents' lives as comfortable and fulfilling as they can be. In short, these are not "homes" – they are "housing". As we discuss in more detail in the chapter that follows, many nursing homes are becoming highly technical subacute care facilities where residents need continuous oxygen and ventilator support, as well as medical and nursing treatment to keep them alive. Yet, as they become ever more medically advanced, for their elderly residents they remain unsympathetic, unpleasant living environments.

America needs to put the "home" back into the nursing home. What does this imply? Well, a nursing home should be more like a family home than a hospital, and family type relationships should be fostered, with the nurses' aides and nursing staff like parents, if you like, as well as healthcare professionals, caring for the residents as one would for one's own family members.

In order to provide our nursing homes with staff properly qualified to care for the elderly residents, we should instigate a training program that prepares staff to administer medication, and provide basic treatments and assessment. Less qualified than registered nurses, these workers would be able to provide a more complete service than certified nurses' aides. To complement their work, personal care assistants would be hired to do laundry, clean rooms, transport patients and equipment, make beds and serve meals. Wages for those workers who have completed a year's training should fall between $15 and $20 per hour – far more than a certified nurses' aide can expect to earn in the current climate. Assigning different staff to the immediate care of residents and the simpler manual work of keeping the home clean and orderly would allow caring staff to spend more time with their elderly charges.

Would this be expensive? Well yes, it would. But is it unreasonable to ask that our senior citizens be properly cared for? Many nurses' aides compare the care of dependant elders to the care of babies. Both need more than just being kept clean, dry and fed. They share a strong need for companionship, affection and emotional and physical contact with the caregivers.

In many traditional societies, the elders are the most respected members of society, and the people who take care of them are acknowledged to be performing a useful, valuable task. For all the benefits that citizenship of America brings, this is far from the case here. Young Americans rightly perceive that caring for the old and sick is not a task to which they should aspire. Migrants from other nations, from the most highly qualified physicians to the most humble nurses' aides, have come to the United States. They are the ones who keep our healthcare system functioning, and we are lucky to have them – without their contribution, our network of nursing homes would grind to a halt. However, we can't relax and assume that qualified professionals from other countries will always keep things ticking over. Many may not want to stay indefinitely – especially at the lower rungs of the medical professional, racism is rampant. As their countries develop, openings will appear in their own hospitals and nursing homes. Their presence is a temporary solution to a deeply rooted problem that must be addressed today.

The government knows that our network of hospitals and nursing homes is in crisis. And the government alone has the power to correct the major deficiencies – quite simply, underfunding and understaffing. However, it is reluctant to use any more capital for healthcare, preferring instead to purchase more homeland security, invested in space exploration and increase its military nuclear arsenal. There are no tangible returns on investment in the aged beyond the quality of life of those individuals, and so they are consistently brushed aside. The public knows that it deserves a better healthcare system, and authorities are eager to shift the blame for its inadequacies onto someone else. Rather than admitting to its own role, the government has adopted the policy of pinpointing individual nursing homes and hospitals and holding them up as examples of what has gone wrong – although most of the flaws of such facilities are directly attributable to underfunding.

It seems probable that the lawsuits, the penalties and the leaking of "bad news" stories will continue. As long as dedicated healthcare workers continue to work for low wages and little recognition, their good faith will be abused. Neglect of residents is sometimes caused by individual error or negligence. But most cases of lapses in hygiene and basic care are the result of chronic understaffing. Nurses and nurses' aides do not have time to do everything. Cases of neglect are not dealt with by identifying the problem and doing something to redress it, but by issuing deficiencies, citations and fines to the nursing facilities in question, thus reducing even further the capital that they have to spend on their patients. The money used to defend lawsuits comes from the budgets that should be used in caring for the weak. The only income the nursing homes are free to administer is that allotted for food, wages, and supplies. When Medicare and state funding do not supply enough revenue to pay for the residents' care, cutbacks have to be made, and when lawyers have to be hired to represent nursing facilities, these cutbacks bite even deeper.

Instead of looking for scapegoats to blame, government-appointed survey groups should isolate problems and work with nursing homes to solve them. Nursing homes and the government are currently opposed, instead of working together to improve our senior citizens' quality of life. Why should nursing homes fear a visit from Medicare and state or federal health administration? A more positive approach would see these visits welcomed as opportunities to enhance cooperation.

The elderly of today are the people who gave us life. We should not repay them by sending them to die in facilities that are little more than prisons, where they are provided with their basic needs and no more. We need to create places to live, not spaces in which to die.

My experience has taught me that state and federal government will continue to reduce the revenue available to nursing homes, without ceasing to demand that quality care be provided. The government will monitor healthcare facilities – especially nursing homes – and punish them with fines and citations in order to parade their lack of tolerance for poor care. None of this will improve the situation. So long as the authorities recoup funds by issuing audits and accusations of fraud, money will be taken from the people who need it most. So long as individual people are isolated and blamed, the cycle of abuse and neglect will continue. Residents will still lie in wet beds, unattended for hour upon end, abandoned in their wheelchairs in hallways and day rooms as they wait to die with little human contact other than that with the dedicated nurses who are overworked, under-paid and at constant risk from work related illness.

CHAPTER FIVE:
1973-1981 – INSPECTING AND ADMINISTRATING

My experience of working as a nursing home administrator throughout the 1970s made it became abundantly clear to me that staffing levels were far too low, although most nursing employees were both willing and able. Nurses' aides were assigned up to ten patients during the day shift, and even more in the evenings and nights. Nursing staff and patients alike were frustrated by the home's inability to provide the standard of care it aspired to.

Perhaps because I was young and full of enthusiasm, I took up the fight to have our budget increased, presenting the corporation with a plan whereby we increased the number of private patients and, with the extra revenue, the number of nursing staff. It was hard to convince them, but I managed to win. I left the fight having learned a valuable lesson. In the nursing home culture, beds represent income, not residents, and empty beds represent a monetary loss.

I soon learned that the most important person in establishing the tone of any nursing home is the activity or social director. This is the person whose job it is to be friendly and upbeat, to encourage the residents to take part in social and activity programs. I was lucky, because the home I administered had one of the best in the business. Rose Johnson – now Rose Soucie – was the type of friendly, outgoing person that everyone should have in their life! Regardless of how difficult things were, she was always positive. She had a real talent for smoothing the ruffled feathers of upset residents, families and staff, and we worked well together. She appreciated the fact that I recognized the value of her work, telling me that no one had shown interest before in the activities and programs she planned. The previous administrator, she said, had spent most of his time sitting in the office doing paperwork. My background in management education had taught me that the most efficient managers get to know their staff and developing interpersonal relationships with them, and with the residents. So I conducted daily visits of the facility, and stopped to talk with everyone.

I worked for the Pacific Convalescent Hospital from June 1973 to February 1975, and I remember this period with some pride. I learned a lot, established a good working relationship with the nursing staff and accomplished what I felt were important changes. Our activity program was strong and residents were all up and about every day, instead of every other day, as had been the case before I came. The standard of nursing care improved, and the facility received no deficiency survey during my time there.

During the late sixties and early seventies, Medicare patients received 100 days of coverage. The decision as to who would receive care was left to a group of doctors –a utilization committee – located in the facility, who reviewed the case. It was assumed at that time that Medicare patients admitted to nursing homes from acute hospital settings would be entitled to 100 days of coverage, but, quite quickly, the federal government found that the cost of this level of care was increasing. They dealt with this by redefining the number of days that Medicare paid for. While the law said that Medicare would pay for post-hospital care for as long as the patient needed skilled nursing care, the Medicare program took it upon itself to decide exactly what skilled nursing care was. Although the local doctor reviewed the patients' cases and decided who was to receive Medicare payment, the government could review and override their decision through their representative, a nurse in one of the fiscal intermediary companies who had contracted with the federal government to pay for Medicare inpatient services.

In the nursing home industry, it was immediately clear that patients who needed 100 days of care were now receiving 20 or 30 days of payment, or even less. With the decrease of nursing days paid for by Medicare, revenue in the industry had to be cut. This in turn led to cutbacks in staffing numbers and nursing services. The program was expanding quickly, and costs were not increasing at the same pace. The cost of caring for patients in acute settings was growing, too, and Medicare had to devise new ways of cutting costs. All of this meant that I, and nursing home administrators around the country, often fell short of supplying the service we aspired to, because our facilities just didn't have the requisite funding.

While I strove to provide the best service I could in the home where I worked, important changes were also taking place in my personal life. It was at this time I met my wife-to-be, Jacqueline. Jackie was born in Sydney, Nova Scotia to Roy and Phyllis

1973-1981 – INSPECTING AND ADMINISTRATING

Matheson on July 22, 1939. Roy was one of the workers in the local steel plant. He and Phyllis had a family of four children, of which Jackie is the second. Jackie always favored an aunt who was a nurse, so it was no surprise that, on graduating from high school, she applied to the Sydney City School of Nursing. After studying for three years, she and three classmates applied for nursing jobs in California, and all were accepted at Modesto, California County Hospital in 1961. Not long afterwards, they went to work for a nursing home in the Berkeley Bay area. Jackie's classmates moved back to Sydney, but Jackie had found a mate, and stayed with him in California. They married and had a son, Robert, and moved to Reno, Nevada, where they lived for ten years. During this time Jackie worked as a nurse, firstly in an acute hospital and latterly in a nursing home. The marriage was not a success and after that period, Jackie moved back to the Bay Area of California on her own to seek work. She was referred to my facility, and that is where we met.

Jackie and I were married in 1975. In that year I also changed jobs, moving to the San Jose District office, where I worked as a health facility representative, or HFR. 1974 and 1975 had seen the increase of Medicare and Medicaid certified facilities in California and across the nation generally. To cater for the increase, additional personnel had to be recruited to conduct certified inspections. These were to take place every year, and complaints were to be handled in a timely manner.

Seeing an opportunity to further my knowledge of the industry, I applied to the Department of Health for a position of inspector. As well as providing me, as a newly-wed – and in 1976, the father of an infant son – with a more secure future, this seemed to be the perfect opportunity for me to help other nursing home administrators, and to use my experience in the field in enhancing the inspection services of the Department of Health. I was duly hired and appointed to the California Office in San Jose. I remember turning up at my new job together with four other new employees. We were all young, enthusiastic and eager to make a difference.

My new position was to combine the roles of consultant and inspector. We were to bring nursing home deficiencies to the attention of the owners and administrators, and make suggestions as to how they might improve their care. Our office staff included health consultants with masters degrees, dieticians and physicians.

I had been shocked, on entering the first nursing home where I worked, by the offensive smell of stale urine. During the years in which I worked as an inspector I encountered far worse, as well as meeting many administrators and nurses who honestly provided the best service that they could – often, for little reward.

Our inspections typically lasted for between three and five days. We invariably began by introducing ourselves to the charge nurse, or by presenting ourselves to the administrator or the director of nurses, and asking to be taken on an inspection tour. This would last for two or three hours, and began with a visit to each patient's room where we would watch the resident nurses and nurses' assistants working. Invariably, we found that there were residents who had not had morning care. In other words, they had not been cleaned and assisted to a chair or, if bed-ridden, had their bed linen changed. Many still had breakfast trays in their rooms and residues of food on their persons or surroundings. Many were still lying in cold, wet beds until as late as 11 a.m. Nurses' aides struggled to complete their morning care and make residents presentable before lunch. In many homes, activities were available from 10 a.m., and while there were usually a few residents taking part, others were left unattended for hours in hallways and dayrooms. Lunch was served hot but was usually cold by the time residents ate it, as the nurses were too busy to help.

Nursing home conditions have changed little since then. While there are horrifying incidents perpetrated by violent, dangerous individuals, most abuse and neglect is caused by understaffing and a lack of qualified supervision. Blame for this situation lies at the feet of the general public, as well as government and administration. We must ask ourselves what level of care is acceptable. What do we want for our parents, and for ourselves, in years to come? We should not accept care levels that are any less than what we aspire to for ourselves.

During the years of my tenure at the Department of Health, I also entered a Masters program in public administration at California State University at Hayward. The department I worked for began to shift its emphasis away from helping nursing homes to improve, towards becoming an enforcement agency with the power to issue fines and citations leading to financial hardship, in the hope of forcing nursing homes to comply. At the same time, the course of study that I was following took the position that humanizing public organizations is the most effective way to make them work for the public good. We were taught that public organizations should strengthen their capacities for intelligent policy analysis and effective action. Administrators should be encouraged to embrace learning, creativity and innovation. It was hard to recognize the wisdom of this approach, and reconcile it with the reality of a healthcare system that was heading towards an enforcement policy of hitting facilities hard and often – to frighten them into submission rather than encourage them to improve.

My studies, which lasted for two years, combined the teachings of sociology, anthropology, philosophy, psychology and economic and organizational studies. We examined social interaction to help us build the tools that would make us more effective leaders. All of this fostered in us a sense of social purpose, the desire to work towards change for the better. I, together with many others, found myself in conflict with the government's approach to the nursing homes' problems in providing high standards of living and quality of life to their residents. It was painfully clear that, through the Medicare and Medicaid programs, the government was both directly and indirectly making price control more important that the quality of care. Their actions reduced competition, fostered poor care and effectively halted innovation and social reform.

As I became more experienced, I saw nursing homes react to government policy by improving the quality of their paperwork and documentation. They grew ever better at justifying bedsores and malnutrition in terms of the medical condition of the patients rather than the quality of their care. They knew that if their paperwork was adequate they would not be penalized! The real problem of the quality of care was not addressed, while the industry and the inspectors remained at loggerheads over documentation and monitoring systems. It was also clear that, with the financial constraints that they were under, even the best nursing homes were struggling. The cost of goods and supplies increased steadily, and the collection of public monies for services given was always late. Medicare and Medicaid both have systems in place preventing the reimbursement of facilities that issued claims late. They can also refuse to reimburse for medical treatment given by deeming it medically unnecessary – even if it was ordered by the patient's own physician!

As the years passed, many of us become gradually more and more uneasy about the direction towards a strict enforcement model with increased citations and fines that the department was taking. Most of us were healthcare professionals, and we were reluctant to find ourselves redefined as police. Quite a number began to seek positions in other areas of government, while others prepared to leave and return to private work as nurses and administrators. I reached the same conclusion in 1981, when I realized that the time had come to move away from working as an inspector. I was thirty-eight years old at that stage – still young, and eager to advance in my chosen profession. Jackie and I dreamt of becoming our own bosses, able to pay our bills and enjoy a reasonable standard of living, while providing quality care to the residents of our nursing home. Fortunately, an opportunity to become independent soon appeared on the horizon.

CHAPTER SIX: SUBACUTE CARE AND THE NURSING HOME

Subacute care is a relatively new system of caregiving that has become an important aspect of healthcare, and one that will continue to grow in importance for the foreseeable future. Seriously ill patients whose conditions have stabilized, but who are not well enough to move to an ordinary nursing home or to their own homes can be taken care of in a skilled nursing facility that provides the technology of a hospital in a nursing home environment. Conditions typically treated in subacute care facilities include brain and spinal cord injuries, neurological and respiratory problems, cancer, strokes, AIDS, and head trauma. Residents suffering from these conditions need more than just simple nursing, but do not always require the intensive, expensive care provided by a hospital.

The American Healthcare Association (AHCA), the Joint Commission on Accreditation of Healthcare Organizations (JCAHO), and the Association of Hospital-Based Skilled Nursing Facilities have developed a definition of subacute care, as follows:

Subacute care is comprehensive inpatient care designed for someone who has an acute illness, injury, or exacerbation of a disease process. It is goal oriented treatment rendered immediately after, or instead of, acute hospitalization to treat one or more specific active complex medical conditions or to administer one or more technically complex treatments, in the context of a person's underlying long-term conditions and overall situation.

Generally, the individual's condition is such that the care does not depend heavily on high-technology monitoring or complex diagnostic procedures. Subacute care requires the coordinated services of an interdisciplinary team including physicians, nurses, and other relevant professional disciplines, who are trained and knowledgeable to assess and manage these specific conditions and perform the necessary procedures. Subacute care is given as part of a specifically defined program, regardless of the site.

Subacute care is generally more intensive than traditional nursing facility care and less than acute care. It requires frequent (daily to weekly) recurrent patient assessment and review of the clinical course and treatment plan for a limited (several days to several months) time period, until the condition is stabilized or a predetermined treatment course is completed.

Although providing subacute care is very different from providing ordinary nursing home care, the same key issue is the root of the problems: understaffing. Subacute care is comprehensive, inpatient care designed for persons who are seriously ill or injured, presenting complex clinical conditions. It must, therefore, be administered by the coordinated services of an interdisciplinary team that includes physicians, nurses, pharmacists and other health professionals, who are trained and knowledgeable in assessing and managing the various conditions. The following are only some of the treatments that must be available: infusion therapy; total parenteral nutrition; ventilation/respiratory care support; orthopedic rehabilitation interventions; post-trauma or CVA therapies; hospice care; specialized Acquired Immune Deficiency Syndrome-related treatments; psychopharmacologic support.

When nursing homes are transformed into technical units, they should increase their staffing hours and install inline continuous oxygen and suction systems. The nursing home will add medical equipment to provide ventilator support and handle medical and nursing treatment. Every subacute unit must have a director, a registered nurse with the leadership skills and knowledge requisite for dealing with medical and nursing problems and for recruiting nursing staff to provide the treatment and care necessary to operate life-sustaining equipment such as ventilators, intra-venous drips, medication, respiratory and wound care, dialysis and more. There is a need for nursing staff in much higher numbers. The state of California has established a minimum of six nursing hours per patient for each day of direct nursing care – one registered nurse to every five patients during the sixteen hours of daytime, and one to every ten during the night, plus certified nursing assistants on each shift. These are the minimum standards, but a properly run subacute care unit will include supervisors, directors, a respiratory health and other specialists. In order that a subacute unit care properly for its patients, it must ensure that 10 to 15% are funded by HMOs or private insurance, as these pay up to 20-50% more than government programs and bring essential revenue into the unit. Effectively, private funding bodies subsidize the government payment programs. Even still, nursing facilities offering subacute care struggle constantly to keep costs down. The growth of publicly owned, run for profit post-acute care companies has also encouraged many traditional long-term care providers to providing services for more seriously ill patients, and these always put profit before the quality of service. Medical supplies and equipment are often not used in the quantities they should be, and corners are cut in terms of quality as institutions are forced to buy the cheapest supplies available. Nor is there enough money to attract the most qualified nurses, and units are often staffed almost entirely by foreign workers whose language skills may not be adequate to communicate properly with patients or families. Cultural differences can, through no one's fault, lead to problems in determining and administering the best possible care. Funding is often lacking, too, for providing continuing onsite education – something which is vital in subacute care.

Because these facilities are located in nursing homes and not in fully equipped hospitals, it is often necessary to work with an acute hospital. Medication, X-rays and medical and laboratory support all need to be provided by external sources, and there are often delays in obtaining the necessary help. Physicians are not always present, usually restricting their input to a weekly visit and occasional phone consultations. More often than not, when subacute residents register a change for the worse in residents' conditions, they have to be transferred to the acute hospital for additional tests, where they experience delays in the emergency room. How much better it would be, if physicians could visit and order appropriate treatment!

Staff must also be equipped to handle state and federal requirements regarding the regulation of consultant's visits, the dispensation of pharmaceutical services and the general operation of subacute care facilities. There are quality improvement programs which must be followed, constant issues of problem solving and interprofessional communications, the interdisciplinary care process including participation in resident assessment and care planning, ongoing needs for the education of facility personnel, residents, families and caregivers about care services, the need for information retrieval, literature evaluation and statistical analysis, the assessment and management of nutritional needs, including enteral and parenteral nutrition delivery systems, the management of drug interaction and adverse drug reactions, pain management, wound care and infection control.

Managers of subacute programs don't just ensure that the technical requirements of the patients are met. They must bring together the right inter-professional team to focus on the medical and nursing needs of the patient, in order to work towards enabling their removal from life support systems. Ideally, the patient completes a course of treatment, and reaches a functional level whereby they can return home, receive a lower level of care in a nursing home or return to hospital for corrective surgery. Residents of subacute units require a high ratio of nurses to patients ranging from the minimum level of 6 to the more appropriate 10 or more nursing hours per day, with the constant attention of nurses and respiratory therapists. The level of care required for subacute patients is four or five times that needed for "regular" nursing home residents. Many people requiring subacute care are admitted directly from intensive respiratory units of acute hospitals. The subacute patient is seen every week by their attending physician, and regularly by specialist physicians in the area of respiratory or infectious disease, or by an internist.

Throughout all this, it is essential that nursing staff and managers of subacute units maintain excellent relations with the families of their patients. Good, clear communication is at a premium.

Case Study: Portrait of a Subacute Patient

Subacute patients are a very special category. Although the majority is aged 65 or older, some can be young. One-third are under 65,[26] and as subacute patients include individuals suffering from AIDS related diseases, breathing difficulties and orthopedic complaints, they vary considerably in terms of health needs, age and background. However, they all share the need for much more intensive healthcare than the majority of nursing home residents. Until relatively recently, the majority of subacute patients was cared for in hospital. Increasingly, they are being discharged to the suba-

---

[26] Barnett, Alicia Ault. "Subacute Care: High Tech Nursing Homes" *Report on Long-term Care* January 12, 1994.

cute sections of nursing homes. One such patient is Simon Vonnegut, who, at 55, is one of Alexander Park's youngest residents. Suffering from advanced Multiple Sclerosis, he is in need of constant care.

It is after midnight, and Simon Vonnegut, subacute patient, is finding it hard to sleep. It's only three weeks since he moved here from the local hospital, and it is taking him time to adjust to the new surroundings.

The first symptom of the dreaded disease, Multiple Sclerosis, occurred when, for no apparent reason, Simon started seeing double. He remembers the first time that this happened with bitterness. Before Simon became too ill to work, he was a civil rights lawyer, working with immigrants from poor countries who are often abused in the workplace because of their lack of official papers and, often, a decent education. Seven years ago, he had just successfully defended a client when, upon leaving the work place, his vision suddenly doubled. Every vehicle on the road appeared to him to be two. The incident didn't last for long, but Simon went to the doctor straight away and, after taking part in a number of tests, heard the shattering diagnosis. A disease like Multiple Sclerosis does not affect just the sufferer, it also changes the lives of their family, forever. At 48, Simon's two children were still of school age, and his wife Amy working only part time. Fortunately, he held good health insurance, but even still, he worried about the future for his family as well as himself.

Multiple Sclerosis is still an incurable disease, but in some people it progresses more quickly that in others. Simon researched all the possible treatments, and tried everything but, unfortunately, the disease progressed rapidly, and as time passed he acquired problems with his gait, balance and bladder control and began to suffer from general mental and physical fatigue as well as unstable temperature control, bone infections, sinusitis and difficulties with breathing. For the first six years, Simon was well enough to be cared for at home, with occasional hospital admissions and part-time nursing help. He and Amy sold their three story house and moved to a bungalow equipped for a wheelchair user. Five months ago, Amy was terrified when she awoke to find Simon turning blue and unable to breathe. His lungs had succumbed to the disease, and he had to be rushed to the nearest hospital and attached to a ventilator for assisted respiration. After some time, his condition stabilized and although he was in need of constant care, it was felt that he could move from the hospital to a nursing home based subacute facility. Simon's health will continue to deteriorate gradually until he dies, but he is not in need of costly acute hospital care. The more intimate setting of a nursing home, coupled with the care of staff trained to deal with medically complex patients is a better environment in which to live, and provides a more pleasant setting for the frequent visits he receives from his wife and sons.

Until a year ago, Alexander Park was home exclusively to elderly residents, bound to a nursing home because of age-related problems. In response to the growing trend of discharging subacute patients to nursing homes, a subacute ward for ten people was opened, and specialized nursing staff employed to care for them. The overheads involved in running a subacute facility are considerable. Medically complex patients are extremely vulnerable to secondary infection, and no risks can be taken. Tubes for ventilators must be changed frequently, and every care must be taken to make the patient as comfortable as possible.

Perhaps partly because of Simon's relative youth and the unfairness of a disease like Multiple Sclerosis that affects people apparently at random, he still feels deeply bitter and resentful and is prone to episodes of severe depression, which make it even harder to take care of him. As every nurse knows, a depressed patient is less likely to respond positively to treatment. Simon, always a very social person, needs company and lively conversation, even though it is no longer easy for him to talk. At Alexander Park, no corners are cut in terms of providing nursing staff, and the facility has ensured that there are enough nurses and nurses' aides to guarantee that no patient will be neglected. Nonetheless, patients would benefit from more interpersonal contact.

The directors of Alexander Park, Alison Goodbody and Jason Brothers, are both in their fifties, and each has a family of teenaged children. For these reasons, they identify strongly with Simon and see him as a symbol of what they hope to achieve in their nursing facility. However, it often seems that the government sees nursing homes as a dumping ground for incurably ill patients. It is cheaper to care for these people here than in hospital, but it's not free. The cost of providing for them threatens the future of Alexander Park, using up all the resources intended for expansion and development. Together with other nursing facilities in the state, Alison and Jason are preparing a proposal for congress seeking increased investment in subacute care. The future welfare of Simon and people like him depends largely on their success.

Although there is no general agreement regarding a precise definition of the term "subacute care", it is fair to say that it covers care not formerly provided by nursing homes – a more intensive, expensive healthcare service for patients with more complex medical needs. In order to provide subacute care, facilities need to be equipped with highly specialized resources, and nursing staff trained to administer them. An interdisciplinary approach is necessary, with staff including physicians, registered nurses, case managers, dieticians, rehabilitation specialists, physical therapists and occupational therapists. Care must be provided for people with conditions as diverse as cancer, cardiovascular problems, wounds, a need for ventilator-assisted breathing and more. All nursing homes are, quite rightly, expected to meet health quality standards. The problem is that many are not paid to do so, and are unable to make ends meet, resulting in a less than perfect service for subacute patients. Subacute care is expensive. It requires staffing levels way beyond the minimal state approved level, state of the art equipment, and a complex, interdisciplinary approach to planning and providing care. The National Subacute Care Association (NSCA) recommends that a distinct unit be provided for subacute patients, and that staff should be more highly trained and spend more time with their patients. Nurse staffing levels generally are greater in subacute care settings than in traditional nursing homes, but they do vary according to facility type. By and large, there are more nursing hours by registered nurses, certified nursing assistants and other nursing staff than in traditional nursing homes. Subacute patients require at least seven or eight direct (hands-on) nursing hours per day but may require more, depending on the medical condition from which they are suffering, excluding the administrative and other non-direct nursing care involved in looking after them. Few facilities are able to provide this level of care, although minimum standards and broadly defined quality guidelines have been developed by The Commission of Accreditation of Rehabilitation Facilities (CARF), and The Joint Commission on Accreditation of Healthcare Organizations (JCAHO) has established accreditation standards for subacute care.

In order to fully understand the healthcare crisis, it is important to appreciate the difference between hospital care, ordinary nursing home care, and subacute care – all distinct treatments for differing needs, with equally diverse costing issues.

Working on the Subacute Ward as a Registered Nurse

Working on a subacute ward brings its own difficulties – it is very different from the routine care of most nursing home residents. Joan Ploughman, Registered Nurse, provides us with some background.

"Taking care of patient in a skilled nursing unit, or subacute ward, is not easy. Seriously ill patients need a lot of attention – physical, mental, social and spiritual. Many are completely dependent on the nursing staff for all their physical needs, and have to be attended to with dignity and respect as well as professionalism. We deal with people with a wide range of complex medical problems, seeing patients with severe wounds, respiratory problems and more. The treatments for critical medical conditions are often technically complex, and no risks can be taken with the patient's health. Running and maintaining a subacute ward is expensive, and many nursing homes are really struggling under the strain of providing a proper service.

Like everyone, subacute patients have their good days and their bad days. Most are unable to communicate with us properly, and it takes a lot of perception to be able to understand their needs, beyond the basic physical care they all receive. Of course, every subacute ward has its success stories which keep us going! So many subacute patients never fully recover, that every happy ending gives the nursing staff a reason to continue.

With subacute patients, we find that their families are often under a great deal of stress, and can become angry with medical staff if they feel that their parent or relative is not being taken care of properly. Most frequently, their concerns are due to misunderstandings. It's important that nursing staff have time to sit and talk with the families about the treatments that the patients are receiving, and explain everything to them in a way they'll understand. Because so many patients have been transferred from an acute ward in a hospital, families sometimes expect them to continue receiving exactly the same treatment, while subacute facilities take care of patients in a slightly less intensive way."

Paying for Subacute Care

The "half way" measure that subacute care represents is seen by many as an important means of reducing healthcare costs, without reducing the quality of attention received by the patient, and many nursing facilities have started to offer this level of care. Many independent studies indicate that moving patients from hospitals into subacute care facilities will dramatically reduce the cost of providing them with medical attention – overall costs for funding the patients' needs could be cut by as much as 50%. The nursing home's overheads, however, will have to increase if they are to provide the help that the patients need. So far, funding levels to nursing homes have not grown as their services have expanded and enlarged, causing these facilities to run the risk of becoming bankrupt and being forced to close. The federal government has failed to adopt a general definition of subacute care, and nor has it developed a system of payments designed to cater for subacute care providers' requirements. The primary payers for subacute care are Medicare and private insurance, with Medicare paying the larger part – around 68% and 22% respectively.

The potential of subacute nursing facilities is huge, both in terms of the type of attention the patients can expect to receive, and of the level of savings the government can make. Once again, however, some investment needs to be made at the outset. If subacute facilities do not receive adequate compensation, they will go bankrupt, and if they go bankrupt, subacute patients will be forced to return to hospitals, where their care is much more costly. Increased Medicare spending on these patients will ultimately reduce the overall cost in providing for their needs, by keeping them out of hospital and in special nursing facilities. This process should include moving resources from acute hospital wards to post acute hospitals and/or subacute care facilities. As the situation currently stands, nursing homes everywhere are experiencing the need to care for patients at a higher acuity level, although many are neither equipped nor staffed to do so. Directors of nurses and nurses do not want to see their charges abused or neglected, but without the necessary resources and personnel, this sometimes cannot be helped. Revenue must increase. The elderly or otherwise incapacitated patients deserve it, their families deserve it, and the people employed to care for them deserve it. Expectations for nursing care are high – and they should be. I have administered nursing homes for more than two decades and it has been my experience that, regardless of how hard we have striven to provide the best service for our patients, no matter how much time is devoted to staff training and to making the caring environment both professional and home-like, our service has always fallen short of our aspirations. In the case of patients in my nursing home who are funded by HMOs and insurance companies, resources have been sufficient to pay for their needs. The situation facing Medicare patients is different, and staffing levels are below the accepted ideal.

The bottom line is that the American taxpayer is not prepared to pay for the level of care that is necessary for the nation's most vulnerable members, and that American politicians are not prepared to anger the taxpayers. Sadly, most people do not fully understand the degree of crisis that prevails until they or their loved ones are in the position of needing care. The taxpaying public, in general, pays without questioning for cars and luxury goods, accepts the need to file tax returns and lawsuits, and to pay for plumbers and decorators to care for their home. When it comes to health coverage, however, the most common attitude is that it should be taken care of by someone else – by the government, by insurance companies, or by health management organizations. Insurance companies and managed health organizations, however, do not really exist for the sake of their contributors – they are businesses, and their purpose is to generate profits for their investors. This they do by cutting corners and restricting services, resulting in a situation whereby money simply does not reach the people who need it most, and increases in funding for healthcare staples, staffing and training are invariably inadequate. Despite Medicare's claim that untold millions are spend on healthcare, it's easy to see that this money is not going where it should – towards increasing staffing and support in caring for our senior citizens. Medicare's payment system is a prospective payment system – reimbursing homes on a "flat rate" basis. This situation creates a compelling financial incentive for nursing homes to reduce the costs of caring for both traditional nursing home patients and sub-acute patients.

There are, quite simply, not enough healthcare workers to provide patients with the attention they need. As the population levels of nursing homes increase – which is inevitable – staffing levels must also increase. Otherwise abuse and neglect will occur, not because nurses and nurses' aides do not want to do their best, but because they cannot. They, too, are victims of Medicare's inadequacies.

Too much emphasis is placed, in certain circles, on subacute care's potential to reduce overall health costs. The effect of this is to keep reimbursement to homes at an impossibly low level, as government administrators create administrative impediments in their payment system, designed to shift the extra cost of caring for subacute patients onto others.

Can subacute nursing facilities be made to work? I believe they can, but the approach – on the part of federal and state government and of healthcare providers – must be realistic. Currently, while hospitals and nursing facility subacute units provide exactly the same treatment to patients, hospitals are awarded higher levels of reimbursement. Nursing facility subacute units must be reimbursed fairly. A new Medicare prospective payment system must be implemented, to provide proper reimbursement for subacute care, and such provision should be made in every state in the country.

CHAPTER SEVEN: GOING SOLO

In 1981, a 70 bed nursing home became available for sublease in San Leandro, California, and Jackie and I took it on, although we had no capital, and had recently acquired a new home of our own in Union City (I withdrew money from my state retirement plan to make payments). Jackie continued to work elsewhere as a nursing director during the first year of the enterprise, while I administered the new business. The facility was not in good condition, and getting it up to standard was a difficult task, although with increased staffing levels, significant improvements were made within a year and Jackie was able to leave her outside job and work in the family business.

Over the years, I had become familiar with many nursing home terms that never ceased to seem offensive. The term "feeding" has to be the worst. Most nurses' aides don't serve residents their meals – they *feed* them as though they were pigs or chickens. Time is of the essence, and the food is forced in as quickly and efficiently as possible. Other terms used to discuss residents that horrify me are the words "up" and "down" when used to describing the process of helping people in and out of bed. When I became owner of St. Luke's convalescent hospital on July 1st, 1981, I resolved that these terms would not be used in my establishment, and that the attitude that accompanies them would have to be stamped out.

The first day of my ownership coincided with the holiday of the fourth of July. Staffing was even shorter than usual and there was no licensed nurse to work. There was only one nurses' aide for every ten patients during the day, and just one licensed nurse for all 70 residents! The nurses were overworked. They were glad to have a new manager, hoping that things would improve. Despite the stress they were under, they were a dedicated staff, and many of the nurses' aides had been employed at the facility for several years. The first step I took was to increase the number of aides on each shift, and inform the staff that our top priority was to provide the best care we could with the resources we had. Once again, one of the first things we had to do was work to eliminate the offensive odor with which I had become so familiar. Many of the nursing staff didn't believe that that would be possible, but it was.

As the husband of a registered nurse, familiar with her problems as director of nurses in private nursing facilities, I had some insight into the working lives of the qualified nursing staff. As soon as the number of nurses' aides in our employ had reached an acceptable level, we began to hire more licensed nurses. The first one we took on still works for us today. She was hired as a licensed vocational nurse, completed her training as a registered nurse several years later and is now the director of nurses.

Economically speaking, the only way that we could continue to improve the quality of care and of life in our nursing facility was to increase revenue. To do so, we began admitting Medicare patients in need of more intensive services and therapy than are usually available in a nursing home. As we increased cost and the range of services available we began to receive more money from Medicare. The quality of care improved, the number of staff members increased, and we were soon able to increase the private population, too.

Costs to Medicare from acute hospitals increased dramatically in the early part of the 1980s, and in response the new prospective payment system was developed and implemented. This would determine the average cost of care for a specific diagnosis, and assign an invariable dollar payment to the service. This new system was implemented over a period of three or four years, beginning in 1983. Prices were held artificially low by the implementation of the new regulations. These controls have had a seriously detrimental effect on the nursing home industry, restricting innovation, fostering social unrest and lowering the quality of both medical care and life, while enhancing the power of the bureaucrats immeasurably. While price control gives the impression of reducing the cost of medical care, what it actually does is reduce the *quality* of medical care, especially in nursing homes where residents are particularly vulnerable. During these years nursing homes all over America struggled to cope with low payment rates. Most managed to provide a minimum standard of care, ensuring that the patients' most basic requirements were met – bathing, feeding and personal hygiene. In our facility, residents were taken out of bed every day, changed every two hours and offered activities. The activity leader had a schedule of events, and documented attendance and the reasons why certain residents did not attend. Medication was ordered in a timely manner and given to the resident, and medical records were reviewed to determine when a physician should be called.

Now, we work with over thirty licensed nurses and sixty nurses' aides, and the quality of care we give has improved enormously since the time when we took over the home. This didn't happen overnight – it takes time to build a workforce, and to pay for it the population of the home had to change. When I took over, most of the residents were beneficiaries of Medicaid, and the home was operating on a very low budget indeed. To increase revenue, we began to accept more private patients. The decisions we made at this time were very much the decisions that were being taken by nursing home administrators and owners all over the country. Like them, we were to continue to feel the pressure of cutbacks in the years to come.

CHAPTER EIGHT: WHEN THINGS GO BADLY WRONG

When confronted with the reality of chronic illness and disability, we would like to believe that our institutions provide humane treatment for the ill and dying. Although that is true for some fortunate individuals who live in high-quality nursing homes, many residents are living in deplorable conditions where they experience painful and unnecessary death. (Christine Harrington, 19th annual Helen Nahm Research Lecture)

Researchers for the United States department of Health and Human Services have identified the principal categories of abuse of nursing home residents. These are: physical abuse, or the infliction of physical pain or injury; the misuse of physical or chemical restraints for controlling a patient, whether beyond the realm of the physician's order or that of established medical practice; verbal or emotional abuse; physical, medical or emotional neglect; the abuse of personal property.

Despite funding studies which show what nursing home residents and their families already know, both government and society have come to accept a standard of care far below that which should be accepted. The standard of care is measured in terms of living conditions, freedom from harm and timely medical treatment. These are all crucial elements. What is not a subject of scrutiny, however, is the official means of documenting conditions in individual homes, and ensuring that criteria are met. As long as nursing homes are able to provide documentation which explains, according to the regulations of the authorities, the reason for apparent neglect or abuse, cases are not investigated. Effectively, checks are made on nursing home's written records, and not on their behavior. The onus on the home is to fulfill demands for clear documentation, not to take excellent care of residents. Thus, care and treatment may be documented without necessarily being provided.

Much abuse and neglect is caused by low staffing levels and a shortage of nurses' aides and licensed nurses. Often, the resident becomes responsible for ensuring his or her own welfare, by making demands and issuing complaints. But not all residents are in a position to say what they need, or to complain if they are mistreated. And it is the nature of nursing homes that residents' conditions deteriorate, through a combination of the inevitable factors of old age, and the lack of help in maintaining the flexibility of aged muscles. The resident who is unable to visit the bathroom without help will soon become incontinent when this help is not forthcoming.

Abuse and Neglect – What's the Difference?

In the legal sense, the term "neglect" – in the context of the nursing home – is used to refer to the failure of those responsible for dependants to exercise a reasonable degree of care. Authorities know that neglect is rampant in nursing homes, and they deal with this by setting standards low enough to allow most nursing homes to reach them. For example, nursing home protocol may dictate that residents be seen every two hours. If, then, the administrators can demonstrate that they are seen that often, neglect is not considered to be present. But what of the resident who needs to take frequent trips to the bathroom? If he or she is left unattended for an hour or more in a wet bed or diaper, isn't this neglect? Officially speaking, no. Not if the rules say that that person need only be seen every two hours.

The law considers as neglect the following: failure to assist in personal hygiene, or in the provision of food, clothing or shelter; failure to provide medical care for physical and mental health needs; failure to protect from health and safety hazards; failure to prevent malnutrition. Because most of the corporate-owned nursing homes are insufficiently staffed, they are unable to provide all the care listed on the residents' care plans and as a consequence, people are often left lying in urine and feces, develop painful, dangerous pressure sores, are not fed properly or given enough to drink, are given too much or too little medication, are dropped, causing bruises or fractures, left unwashed and ungroomed, ignored and left in bed all day.

The Situation Today

Many nursing homes are now run by corporate entities, which administer chains of establishments. While some of these provide excellent care, many are noteworthy for their lack of personal attention, and their reduction of patients' needs to the bottom line –

cost. The conditions that prevail in some of these nursing homes beggar belief, but because they have the financial and political clout to resist criticism, they often go unpunished.

One scandal, reported in 1999, [27] occurred when the State Governor, Gray Davis, included the president of a nursing home company with thirty homes with a history of fraud and even mistreatment of residents, on an overseas trade mission. Earlier, the company, Horizon West, had settled a Medicare fraud claim which included accusations of billing for luxury items such as wine and designer shoes. The company had also been accused of negligence when one resident with a history of choking died after she choked on her food.

In ideal circumstances, the Medicare/Medicaid system of benefits would serve to equalize the treatment given to wealthier and poorer patients. In fact, because nursing homes make less money from Medicare patients, some actively discriminate against them, as in the case of a Tampa nursing home, which, in 1998, discharged its Medicare residents. [28]

It was time to lay carpeting and hang wallpaper, the nursing home said, so dozens of elderly and bedridden residents had 30 days to move out with no guarantee that they could return. It was just a coincidence, the home's owners said, that all the patients evicted were on Medicaid and that the building had been renovated three months earlier. But in a coincidence involving the operators' parent company, Vencor, news of the evictions came the same day Vencor's top executive was quoted in The Wall Street Journal as saying that the company planned to rid its nursing homes of Medicaid patients, who bring in less money than private patients.

Now Florida is investigating whether the $3.5 billion nursing home giant tried to dump Medicaid patients using the renovation project as a ruse.

Unlike most nursing homes in Florida, Vencor's Rehabilitation and Healthcare Center of Tampa is not required to accept a certain number of Medicaid patients for state licensing. That means a wholesale Medicaid eviction would be "not necessarily illegal but ruthless," spokeswoman Edie Ousley of the state

---

[27] Pyle, Amy, Los Angeles Times, Monday, November 8, 1999.

[28] Chicago Tribune, Thursday, April 9, 1998.

Agency for Healthcare Administration said Wednesday. So the investigation will also focus on the quality of care at the home, she said. The state launched an investigation of Vencor's 20 other Florida nursing homes, which have about 2,000 Medicaid beds in all. Eleven of the homes are required under their state licenses to accept Medicaid patients. "They were moving them out so quickly. These patients were crying, 'Where are we going to go?' They were being treated like cattle being herded," said Nelson Mongiovi, whose 93-year-old mother was among the 52 patients ordered discharged. Mongiovi was named a plaintiff in an emergency injunction issued ... to halt the discharges and was listed as plaintiff in a lawsuit expected to be filed Thursday against the nursing home. A spokeswoman for Vencor, based in Louisville, KY., said the court action was unnecessary because the nursing home agreed to halt the discharges once it realized the state was concerned. "We wanted to do what's most sensitive for the patients," said Susan Moss. Moss said it was a coincidence that the patients ordered discharged were all Medicaid patients. The discharges were needed because the 170-bed home was under going the second phase of a renovation project, she said. The state was particularly concerned because on the day officials learned of the discharges, the Journal published an article about Vencor evicting all Medicaid patients from an Indianapolis home and making plans to withdraw homes in nine states from Medicaid. "We'll go out of Medicaid in all 300 buildings if we don't start see a little change in the Medicaid program," Chief Operating Officer Michael Barr told the newspapers.

The internationally respected magazine, Time [29] also depicted alarming scenes of abuse in American nursing facilities, focusing on homes in California. Reporter Mark Thompson spoke to the relatives of elderly nursing home residents who suffered appallingly at the hands of those paid to care for them, detailing incidents of beating, malnutrition, dehydration and neglect. In one case, an aged patient, who entered a "convalescent hospital" with a degenerative brain disease, also suffered bruises, bedsores and a broken pelvis within months of her admission. Her death was attributed to choking on food, although the patient in question was supposed to be fed through a tube. Following the publicity instigated by this patient's daughter, some former employees of abusive nursing homes came forward to testify. Their reports of mistreatment of elders, and systematic misrepresentation of working and living conditions to the authorities make chilling reading, including the

---

[29] Mark Thompson, "Shining a Light on Abuse", Time, August 3rd, 1998.

failure to change a bandage for nearly two weeks, preventing residents from finishing their meals, and patients developing bedsores to the bone because they were not moved often enough.

In many cases, patient neglect would be prevented by increasing staffing levels, [30] but federal government has passed no law that makes provision for minimum numbers of nurses and nurses' aides, facilitating corner-cutting by unscrupulous nursing home owners. Even in homes which genuinely strive to do their best for patients, inadequate funding often prevents administrators from being able to hire sufficient numbers of staff.

Quite apart from their frequent shortcomings, care facilities that depend upon the Medicare/Medicaid system of benefits suffer a logistical nightmare, which sees nursing and other medical staff reduced to spending their working hours trying to balance books instead of doing what they are trained for. In the words of one healthcare worker: "We are forced to sit behind a desk and push paper instead of being out on the floor in the room taking care of the people that we are in this industry for in the first place. The paperwork is never-ending, and it is only getting worse."Another important issue in protecting the well being of nursing homes' elderly residents is that of ensuring that the people hired to care for them will not do anything to harm them. Of course, most healthcare workers are dedicated professionals. However, there is always a small risk that individuals who, for whatever reason, feel compelled towards violence or other criminal acts, might apply for work in a nursing facility. For this reason, it is important to check the backgrounds of all such applicants. As the situation stands, nursing facilities are unable to check the registries of states other than their own, allowing nurses' assistants with criminal or otherwise violent records to move from state to state and, in a worst-case scenario, to hurt, steal from or abuse their wards. Again, the arguments against such a centralized system boil down to one basic component: cost. It is not cheap to set up and maintain an information network of the type that I have just described. Again, one must look to the long rather than the short-term. Investment in such a

---

[30] Jones JS. Elder abuse and neglect: understanding the causes and potential risk factors. Am. J. Emerg. Med. 1997 Oct; 15(6); 579-83.

procedure at this point in time will result in less waste later, in minimizing the risk of exposing vulnerable elderly, sick or disabled people to "carers" with a tendency to injure or steal. This is a practical issue – and it is also one about basic human rights. Abuse has taken place in nursing homes, ranging from sexual assault to minor pilfering. It continues to occur, and with low staffing levels, can go undetected for some time.

CBS news also made the following grim assessment of the situation [31]

They are about the last places anyone wants to be, but about 1.6 million people now live in nursing homes in the United States. Thirty years from now, it's expected to be 5 million.

Many patients are at risk because one out of four nursing homes every year is cited for causing death or serious injury to a resident, according to government figures.

Alice Oshatz is looking for an assisted living facility because at 85 she could no longer live alone, and she won't move in with her children. "I never thought this could possibly happen to me," she said. When she was asked if she's worried about becoming a burden, Oshatz began to cry. "Yes, oh yes. That's the really hard part of it. My daughter lovingly she does it and everything, but I don't want, if I'm going down, to pull her down," she added. The family is agonizing over Oshatz's decision to move into an assisted-living home where she would still have a fairly independent lifestyle. But Oshatz is already thinking about the day when she may need a lot more care, and like half of elderly Americans she may have to move into a nursing home. That's an idea she dreads. "I hope I go quietly into the far beyond," said Oshatz. She is not the only one who feels that way. Eighty-three percent of elderly Americans would stay in their homes until the end if they could. Thirty percent say they'd rather die than go into a nursing home. And their fears may be well founded. Nursing home inspection documents show that more than a quarter of American nursing homes were repeatedly cited for serious violations that caused death or injury to patients. In California, a third of the homes have been cited for

---

[31] Vince Gonzalez, CBS news.

WHEN THINGS GO BADLY WRONG

causing serious harm or death to patients. In 1998, less than 2 percent of California nursing homes had no violations.

A CBS News analysis of the federal government's nursing home inspection database finds more than 1,000 homes were cited last year for hiring staff with a history of abuse. Federal regulators admit, however, that the statistics conceal how bad things really are inside America's nursing homes. State inspections are often unreliable, and most problems in nursing homes go unreported. That's especially true when it comes to cases of physical abuse.

"Elder abuse is fast becoming one of the greatest law enforcement challenges of the next century," said Paul Hodge who investigates crimes against the elderly. The Love family knows this all too well. As a veteran of three wars, Donald Love was buried with full military honors at Arlington National Cemetery. But it was his wife, Helen, who was wounded in battle, at age 75. Bruce Love found out his 75-year-old mother had been attacked by a nursing home staff member only after he called to check on her. But the home told him not to worry; everything was fine. He said he was told "that there wasn't any problem, that she'd been examined by a doctor, and there weren't any major injuries." And according to the nursing home doctor's report, "There was no head injury. No loss of consciousness ... X-rays do not disclose any fracture of the mandible, forearm or wrist." The doctor said any bruising Love had was caused by her "medical illnesses." Bruce's brother Gary reached his mother's side first. "I couldn't believe what I was seeing, bruises on her neck, on her chin," he said. "She had some bruises on her legs. I said, 'What the hell happened to you here?'" He wanted to take his mother to a hospital emergency room a block or so away but the home refused to release her. Gary Love said it was only after he threatened to call police that administrators backed down.

"I couldn't touch her because they hadn't substantiated what her injuries were. This is in the hospital emergency room with my mother laying on a gurney, and I could not comfort her," said Bruce Love. Emergency room doctors quickly discovered that despite what the nursing home said, Helen Love had a dislocated neck and a broken wrist. She was covered with bruises. Her condition was so grave doctors were afraid to operate on her neck. Instead they drilled holes in her skull and fitted her with a steel halo to hold her head up. It was a painful and draining treatment. So what exactly happened to Helen Love? On the night she was attacked, the 95-pound woman was bedridden in room 8B of the Valley Skilled Nursing Home in Sacramento, Calif. Around 7 p.m. on his eighth day on the job, certified nurse's assistant Tim Saeleeentered

The Crisis in America's Nursing Homes

Love's room and found that Love had soiled herself and needed cleaning. That upset Saelee, and he began handling her roughly. When she complained, Saelee attacked her, an eyewitness – and Love herself – told police.

"He got real ferocious and started beating me all around the bed," said Helen Love. "He choked me and went and broke my neck ... and broke my wrist," she said. Love decided the only way she could survive was to play dead. Eventually Saelee left her room.

"I was going to fight ... And I'm black and blue all over," said Helen Love.

When asked if she tried to fight back, she said, "Oh, I'm not a quitter; I'm a fighter. But two days after she was interviewed on videotape, Helen Love died.

"I honestly feel that I let her down. I still feel that today. And that's what's so frustrating about this," said Bruce Love.

Also frustrating for the Love brothers is the sentence that the nurse's assistant received for attacking their mother.

"He did plead guilty to elder abuse, which got him a year in the county jail. You can go out on the street as an innocent person and have boxing match with somebody you don't like and get more time for simple assault or tax evasion!" said Bruce Love.

And this was not the first time Saelee was accused of abuse. He had been warned about rough handling of patients at another Sacramento nursing home. Then he was fired for threatening to hit a resident.

He was hired a month later at Valley Skilled. At this facility three other employees had convictions for abuse, which under state law should have prohibited them from working in a nursing home.

No one at the home would talk to CBS News on camera because the Love family is suing.

"I don't ever want to see another person ever have this done to them," said Bruce Love.

Company lawyers told CBS News that what happened was not the home's fault. It did everything the law required. But clearly in this case and across the nation, dangerous nursing home workers are not being detected, and elderly people certainly aren't being protected.

At least 33 states do some kind of background check on a very small number of nursing home workers but none require a national background check. And a recent government report found state background checks aren't working, saying,

"There was no assurance that individuals who may pose a risk to residents are systematically identified and barred from nursing home employment."

The California Department of Health Services told CBS News that it has revoked the license of one nurse assistant at the Valley Skilled Nursing Home.

Officials are also checking licenses of all nurses and nurse assistants at the home and are referring the case to the California Attorney General's Office.

Valley Skilled Nursing Home's parent company, North American Healthcare runs 17 facilities in California and applied to open three more homes in California but were turned down by the state in September 1999 because of "consistently poor care" in their facilities.

A recent article from the Kansas City Star [32] outlines abuse in nursing homes in horrifying detail, and highlights the importance of keeping staffing at an acceptable level. (The emphasis in the quotation that follows is mine):

Workers at Claywest House said they had warned their supervisors that Karl Willard, an aide at the St. Charles, Mo., nursing home, tormented elderly residents.

But the 180-bed nursing home was shorthanded and Willard stayed on the job.

Not long after that warning two years ago, one of Willard's patients died of a head injury. A grand jury indicted Willard and in February, he pleaded no contest to first-degree elder abuse for the death of Marshall Rhodes, 78.

In lawsuits filed after Rhodes' death, his family and others alleged Claywest House didn't have sufficient staff.

Rhodes' family settled for an undisclosed amount. In March, Claywest and its management company, American Healthcare Management, settled six other

---

[32] Joe Lamb, The Kansas City Star, 05/06/2000.

lawsuits alleging mistreatment for nearly $2.5 million. The home and management company admitted no wrongdoing.

Charles Kaiser, president of American Healthcare Management, said that the home has sometimes had problems finding workers but that it today is a good facility in good standing and "humming along just fine."

Staffing problems are not unusual in nursing homes, according to a recent study by the Institute of Medicine, a national research group. At a time when people 85 years of age and older are the fastest growing segment of the U.S. population, there is a critical nationwide shortage of healthcare workers.

In Kansas, Connie Hubbell, the state's secretary of the Department of Aging, said staff shortages and high turnover rates at nursing homes also are a problem. So far, Hubbell said, homes have been able to meet minimum staffing needs without an upsurge in complaints.

But that's not the case in Missouri, where staffing problems contributed to a 21 percent increase in the total number of complaints against nursing homes in 1998 and 1999 combined, the latest years for which data are available.

Richard Dunn, director of the state's Division of Aging, said staff shortages are threatening the quality of care for America's old and infirm. Dunn's advice for nursing homes: "Don't admit them (patients) if you can't take care of them. We can't justify poor quality care because of staff shortages."

What's more, homes desperate to find staff sometimes are not doing enough to screen out potentially dangerous workers, according to the national study and Missouri auditors.

Legislators in the Missouri House recently passed a bill to prevent nursing homes from hiring people listed as unfit to work with children or the mentally ill. The bill is pending in the state Senate, where it failed last year. […]

Advocates of legislation pending in Missouri say there is a special urgency to fixing staffing and other problems in nursing homes. Within the next five years, the number of Missouri residents 60 years of age and older will increase from 950,000 to 2 million, Dunn said.

And the first wave of the baby boomer generation will turn 65 in 2011.

As more people get older, more nursing home problems are ending up in court. And because of more lawsuits, liability insurance costs for Missouri homes increased 500 percent or more in the past year, Carlson said.

In lawsuits involving Claywest House, families of six former patients contended that staff shortages led to poor, negligent or abusive care. Among the allegations:

- Failure to feed or give water to a resident who later died.
- Locking away the cane of a resident who later suffered a broken hip and died from complications.
- Allowing ants to infest a resident.

Kaiser, president of American Healthcare Management, said the lawsuits amount to only allegations. The home and the management company admitted no wrongdoing in the settlements.

Kaiser said that nursing homes throughout the country need 300,000 nursing aides and that they are hard to find. Claywest even hired people from a Salvation Army shelter, which he said helped the nursing home and the poor.

"That facility (Claywest) deserves an award," Kaiser said.

Kaiser said the lawsuits result from what he called an attorney feeding frenzy that only drives up insurance costs and compounds the problems of caring for the elderly.

Tim Dollar, one of Kansas City lawyers who represented the families, disagreed. "There can't be a lawyer feeding frenzy," Dollar said, "without food in the water."

Jim Bartimus, an attorney who works with Dollar, said such lawsuits force homes to make improvements. If they don't provide good care up front, Bartimus said, lawyers will make them pay more in the end.

Among the plaintiffs in the lawsuits filed against Claywest was Bonnie Thorpe of St. Peters, Mo. Thorpe said she often visited her mother, Edythe Beck, and helped care for her.

But Thorpe had to leave the state on a short trip in May 1999. Then her mother died. A doctor said the cause of death was starvation, dehydration, pneumonia and infection.

Thorpe said that her 74-year-old mother, like many advanced Alzheimer's patients, had to be coaxed to eat and drink. Thorpe said she fed her before leaving on May 16, 1999. According to court records, she later discovered that no one else fed her mother for five days, at which point she died.

Kaiser said patients with advanced Alzheimer's often refuse to eat and die of starvation. He said state law does not allow workers to force feed them.

Another plaintiff, Robert Jones of St. Charles, said his 84-year-old mother needed a cane and her glasses to walk when he put her in the home in August 1999.

Jones said he visited days later and found her cane locked in a nursing cabinet and her glasses in another patient's room. She didn't have them again two days later, he said, when she fell and broke her hip.

When called to the home, Jones said, "I picked her up and put her in a chair and wheeled her to the car and a hospital myself."

According to court papers, she died of complications from the fall on Aug. 25, 1999 -- 23 days after she entered Claywest.

In another case, an 86-year-old woman allegedly left lying in her own waste was found covered with ants. The lawsuit contends that family members picked ants off her days later as she died of natural causes.

Most of the incidents alleged in the lawsuits occurred in 1999. At that time, the state had cited the home for staff shortages and other problems. It was operating on a temporary license.

The Division of Aging proposed more than $360,000 in fines over two years. That ended last fall with a settlement for $128,000 -- the largest such fine ever collected in Missouri.

Today, Claywest is open and in good standing again with the state.

But Thorpe said nursing homes that cannot provide enough staff should not admit patients. Her mother's care, and subsequent death, have left her afraid of her own so-called golden years.

"Anyone of us could end up in that boat," Thorpe said.

Sexual Abuse of Nursing Home Residents

To any reasonable person, sexual abuse is appalling, in all its guises. For most, the sexual assault of an aged, vulnerable nursing home resident is not just appalling, it's unimaginable. Sadly, however, it does occur. Sexual assault takes various forms, with rape being the most commonly reported incident. [33] The following are just two of the many cases brought to public attention in recent years.

Nursing Home Found Liable for Employee's Sexual Assault: 70-Year Old Woman Attacked [34]

WOODBRIDGE, N.J., July 3 /PRNewswire/ -- In one of the first cases brought under a state nursing home residents rights law, a New Jersey elder care facility was found liable for an employee's sexual assault on a 70-year old woman.

Ocean County Superior Court Judge Frank A. Buczynski recently held that Kensington Manor Care Center of Toms River violated the rights of Sybil Watson when certified nurse assistant Edward Argueta shoved his fingers into her vagina at 4:30 a.m. after he told her to go into the bathroom and bend over the sink, where he proceeded to violate her.

Ms. Watson also contends that a similar incident had happened two weeks earlier yet she failed to report it because she felt ashamed.

"Mistreatment and abuse of this sort is disgusting and, unfortunately, a fact of life in nursing homes," said Watson's attorney, Alan M. Darnell, of the Woodbridge, NJ-based law firm Wilentz, Goldman & Spitzer.

"Nationally, more and more cases have been reported where residents have been subjected to inhumane, humiliating, and painful treatment that deny the basic human rights guaranteed to them by this statute," added Darnell.

Darnell won a summary judgment under the Nursing Home Responsibilities and Rights of Residents Act. The court held as a matter of law that Argueta's conduct amounted to a violation of " ... the right to a safe and decent living environment and considerate and respectful care that recognizes the dignity and individuality of the resident."

---

[33] Todd M. Elder Alert. A newsletter for senior concerns from the office of the attorney general. Vol. 6, No. 3, p.1-4.

[34] Newswire, July 3rd, 2001. Source Wilentz, Goldman & Spitzer, P.A. (Founded in 1919, Wilentz, Goldman & Spitzer, P.A. is a full-service law firm with 140 attorneys. The firm has offices in Woodbridge and Eatontown, New Jersey, and New York City.)

Argueta plead guilty to the fourth-degree crime of assault on an institutionalized elderly person. He was sentenced to a noncustodial period of probation, during which he is unable to work as a healthcare provider in the State of New Jersey.

A separate hearing will be conducted to determine damages to be awarded to the victim.

Facility May Be Liable In Sexual Assault By Unsupervised Aide [35]

Victoria Ann Elder's last years were tragic. The victim of an automobile accident, Ms. Elder was a quadriplegic and confined to her bed at the Stone County Skilled Nursing Facility in Mountain View, Arkansas. One Saturday evening the helpless woman was sexually assaulted by an aide at the nursing home.

William McConnaughey, an aide at the facility who had begun his employment as a janitor and taken a two-week course to become a nurse's aide, was assigned to clean and change Ms. Elder. At about 8 p.m. that Saturday another aide observed Mr. McConnaughey molesting Ms. Elder.

The second aide talked to a senior nurse, who told her to "wait to see if it happened again." She knew that was an inadequate answer, and reported what she had seen to the charge nurse.

The charge nurse, in turn, attempted to contact the facility's director of nursing and nurse administrator. Neither was available on Saturday night, but the charge nurse made no effort to file a complaint with the authorities.

Monday morning the charge nurse told the nursing home's management what had happened, and the facility took quick action. After the nurse administrator interviewed witnesses and notified Ms. Elder's father and physician, she contacted the police.

A lawsuit was filed on Ms. Elder's behalf sixteen months later, relying on two separate theories. The first claimed "vicarious" liability for Mr. McConnaughey's actions because they occurred in the course of his employment with the nursing home. The second maintained that the nursing home was liable because it had been negligent in its supervision. The trial judge dismissed Ms. Elder's complaint, finding that the nursing home had no reason to expect that

---

[35] Elder Law Issues, April, 2001, Volume 8, No. 41.

Mr. McConnaughey might molest a patient. Ms. Elder's estate (she died after the lawsuit was begun) appealed.

The Arkansas Court of Appeals agreed with the trial judge on one of the lawsuit's theories, but sent the matter back for trial on the other. Mr. McConnaughey's misbehavior was obviously not within the scope of his duties, the judges decided, and there was no reason for the nursing home to expect he might do such a thing. The nursing home was not directly liable for his actions.

On the subject of the home's supervision of Mr. McConnaughey, on the other hand, the trial judge was wrong. At least one expert witness was prepared to testify that Stone County had a history of failing to supervise aides (based on deficiencies noted in prior facility surveys), and that they permitted male aides unmonitored access to helpless patients. The Court of Appeals ordered a full trial on the negligent supervision claim.

Most nursing homes are unable to run full checks on the criminal records of their staff – some abusers have, incredibly, already been fired from nursing homes for sexual misconduct, and understaffing is so severe that the sexually violent may be able to secure access to patients for long enough to assault them. Imagine the confusion and pain of the resident with Alzheimer's disease, or another type of dementia, or the frustration of the paralyzed, wheelchair bound resident whose Parkinson's disease prevents him or her from speaking out. Sadly, sexual predators form part of our society. I hope that this will not always be the case. In the context of the nursing home or hospital, however, we must take a pragmatic view. So long as chronic understaffing remains the norm in the nursing homes of America, our elders will be vulnerable to opportunistic sexual predators. Staff levels must be increased for many reasons, and this is one of them.

What constitutes sexual abuse in the environment of the nursing home? Effectively, the same criteria that are used anywhere. Sexual abuse is any form of nonconsensual sexual contact, including unwanted or inappropriate touching, rape, sodomy, sexual coercion, sexually explicit photographing and sexual harassment. Not all nursing home residents are in a position to indicate explicitly their consent or lack of consent to sexual contact. In these circumstances, all such contact is abusive.

When sexual abuse is perpetrated against the resident of a nursing home, the abuser is usually an employee of the home. However, understaffing can lead to abuse of one patient by another. Again, pragmatism is in order. Rather than assuming or hoping that such assaults will not take place, we must ensure that staffing levels are such that they cannot. Abusive occurrences have also been noted featuring family members and even strangers who have broken into the nursing facility. We must be realistic; the only way that we can guarantee our elders that they will not be victims of unwelcome, violent sexual attention is by maintaining high staffing levels. Sexually violent people exist in our society, whether we like it or not. They are a small minority, but are capable of causing severe harm. We gain nothing by pretending that they do not exist, and everything by acknowledging this unsavory fact, and by appointing sufficient nursing staff to prevent sexual violence from occurring in nursing homes.

Abuse Generated by the System Itself

Dangerous or negligent individuals cause a great deal of damage in nursing homes, but the very system of administration that has been created by the authorities is abusive. I began my career in the nursing home business as a direct caregiver, and moved on to become, respectively, an administrator, and inspector and, at last, an owner. The journey has taken me thirty years, and to reflect on the history of nursing homes throughout this period is both instructive and painful. There have been few major changes in the way that nursing homes care for the elderly. The biggest shift has been the growing emphasis on uniformity and homogeneity. The layers of regulations generated by the Medicare program and imposed on nursing homes have turned the individual homes' managers into pawns, manipulated by regulations. Policies and procedures are adopted uniformly, with only slight room for adaptation to the peculiar needs of each facility. While no one can dispute the importance of quality control, the current situation has resulted in the impossibility of innovation and thoughtfulness on the part of managers. Innovation is considered undesirable – what is admired is the ability to comply with regulations unquestioningly, and to appease inspectors, making every home's first priority the rules, and not the residents.

Regulations are not written with the elderly in mind. Old people need rules that are adjusted to their needs. Instead, rules require specific things to be done at specific times. Meals must be served when the rules demand it, not when the patients are hungry. The elderly cannot choose when, where or what to eat. Neither do they enjoy much say over their other activities. There is no need for this situation. Nursing homes could easily operate with a system whereby dining areas were open for prolonged periods, and offer a range of meals from a menu. This would allow residents a degree of autonomy. The right to make basic decisions about one's daily activity is a basic, human right, and its absence constitutes an abuse. Similarly, the lack of space available to individual residents violates their right to privacy, as does their inability to decide when to bathe. Medical assistance from a physician should be available when the resident has need of it, and not just when the regulations say it's time for the doctor to make his call.

The regulations that have been put in place to order the lives of the residents of nursing homes are very telling. These are not rules designed to enhance the lives of our fellow citizens, because at many levels of society, the elderly are no longer thought of as fully functioning people. Many elderly people, although physically weak, are mentally alert and capable of making valuable contributions to society. All elderly people, including those who are profoundly confused, have formed part of the weave of social life. Nobody deserves to be locked in a home and subjected to demeaning, belittling rules, but this is what happens when management, nursing home owners, employees, government, families and the public see nursing homes as businesses with products that have to be processed. The fact is, of course, that the "product" is a broken, dependent, needy but still very human person who relies upon others for their comfort and well being. And, of course, well being is about more than just basic hygiene and regular meals.

The dehumanization of the elderly has become so widely accepted, that even the individual's right to live is now questioned. The power of attorney has given permission to withhold life-sustaining treatment and even, in some cases, the withdrawal of food and water to hasten death. There are some instances in which a dignified death is better than a long and painful struggle but it is my view that the deaths of many elderly people are hastened along in a very unseemly manner. Shortening the lives of our nursing home residents in no way addresses the problem.

The government officials responsible for budgetary allocation rarely, if ever, step inside a nursing facility. They have no real idea of how their decisions affect the lives of so many people, and their political spin, together with the ill-conceived Medicare program of today serve only to conceal the reality of nursing facilities.

All over America, nursing facilities contain dedicated, honest nursing staff whose mission it is to care for our elderly. Sadly, however, they are often working side by side with colleagues who are under-trained and ill-equipped to provide the services that are needed. We need more than just compassion from our healthcare workers. We need to encourage innovation in caring for the elderly. Instead of punishing innovators, we should foster their contribution.

Under President Johnson, the United States took its first steps towards providing full healthcare. This was an important development, but times have changed, and so must our healthcare provisions. Government has categorically failed to provide the leadership and direction to lead the industry towards a mature, meaningful future. Iron rules instigate fear in the hearts of nursing home administrators; they do not provide a caring environment in which our elders can spend the remaining years of their lives. Environments are regulated and rules and routines implemented. Owners and healthcare organizations are occupied in simply administering the regulatory functions of the facility, keeping the paperwork up-to-date, conducting daily inspections of the facilities to ensure that equipment and safely areas are in compliance with the regulations. Patient care is in the hands of the director of nurses whose responsibility it is to write schedules and see that treatment and medications are proved. Most directors of nurses have little time to spend with residents, being fully occupied appeasing relatives and attending to office duties.

Understaffing hurts nurses and other healthcare professionals. It also hurts the people they care for. In 1999, the Institute of Medicine published some alarming statistics, which revealed that medical errors cause from 44,000 to 98,000 deaths in hospitals a year. To put that into perspective – medical errors kill more people on a yearly basis than do car accidents, breast cancer or AIDS![36] How many of these occurred because nurses and doctors were allotted more patients than they could care for, were working overtime yet again or were left without the necessary support? Despite the evidence to the contrary, HMOs and other authorities, with their eye on the balance sheet, insisted that these problems did not arise because of understaffing, overtired carers and compulsory overtime, but for other reasons – reasons that did not require investment of cash into the nation's healthcare system. Let's take a look at some of the statistics obtained by the investigative report cited above:

As nurses have less time to spend with their patients, medication errors and other adverse incidents have become a regular occurrence: 34 percent of nurses say that patients on their units experience missed or delayed medication or treatments at least once a week. 8 percent report that the wrong medication or dosage, which can lead to serious complications, is administered to patients on their units at least once a week. 10 percent say that patients on their units acquire infections, which are often the result of delayed medication or treatment, at least once a week ... A majority of nurses identify understaffing as the cause of medical errors. And the situation, they say, is not improving. 54 percent of nurses say that half or more of the errors they report are the direct result of inadequate staffing. Despite the growing attention focused on medical errors, most nurses say the rate of incidents has remained unchanged during the last year — while fully 30 percent of nurses say the errors have actually increased ...

The fact that our nursing home residents come second in importance to the nursing home rules is an abuse in itself. I hope that it will not always be so.

Avoiding Nursing Home Abuse and Neglect

In order to minimize the possibility of the occurrence of abuse or neglect, nursing homes need to implement certain strategies. When each resident is admitted, a plan of care should be developed, tailored to meet that person's needs and discussed in detail with both the resident and the family. The plan should include details of the daily medication and treatment provided, the activity program avail-

---

[36] *The Shortage of Care*, a study by the SEIU Nursing Alliance.

able in the nursing facility and the resident's needs in terms of nursing and medical attention. Currently, however, documentation has become so over-valued that nurses spend more time in writing reports and documentation for authorities than they do in carrying out their nursing duties. Devoting nursing hours to paperwork is the only way in which nursing homes can protect themselves from accusations of neglect and abuse. Ironically, the very paperwork intended to prevent abuse occurring can lead to neglect, as it takes the nurses away from where they are most needed.

Two of the common underlying factors of many illnesses and changes in condition of the elderly are dehydration and malnutrition, which can lead to confusion and dementia. One would think that intake of food and water is easy to monitor, but with low staffing levels, it can be difficult to keep track. As people grow old, their appetites and intake of fluids decline. Without careful attention, this can lead to urinary and liver problems, skin breakdown and overall weakness.

Most abuse can be prevented by taking the simple measure of ensuring reasonable staffing levels in all of our nursing facilities. But is this really going to happen?

CHAPTER NINE: DEALING WITH DIFFERENCE [37]

Racism is far from absent from public life in the United States and unfortunately, racism in the nursing home environment is yet another shortcoming that needs to be addressed. Racism, although it stems from simple prejudice and bigotry, is manifested in complex ways and within nursing facilities, racism can occur towards residents, on the part of residents towards staff, among staff and among residents. The only way to move towards a brighter future is to address this issue realistically – it has been ignored and left unattended for far too long.

Cultural Issues

The most complex form of discrimination is not really racial at all. It is cultural, based on people's ethnically acquired sets of beliefs and approaches to the world. Much cultural discrimination grows, not from bigotry, but from a failure to understand diversity. Different cultural groups have markedly different attitudes towards old age, illness, death, religion and even simple matters such as modesty, personal relationships and family. Cultural differences should always be respected, whether it's a case of avoiding serving non-kosher food to religiously observant Jews, respecting the Hispanic patient's need for the presence of family, or recognizing that the degree of physical intimacy considered appropriate varies greatly from culture to culture – (among people of Anglo-Saxon origin, for example, some distance is generally maintained between individuals, while people from the Middle East tend to stand very close together when they talk. Neither approach is "wrong" – they are just different). In old age, we tend to revert to our cultural roots,

---

[37] Most racism in the context of the nursing home is directed towards Black, Hispanic, American Indian and other minorities, so our focus here is on these groups. However, there have been reports of racism towards white healthcare workers in homes where the majority belongs to another group. It goes without saying that this type of behavior is no less reprehensible. The fact that we cannot cover this issue fully reflects limitations of space, and not a disregard for the details of the issue of racism in the healthcare system.

and it is not uncommon to find elderly people stressing the importance of issues which did not bother them unduly during their younger years.

Of course, most healthcare workers are not social anthropologists too, and we can't expect them to immediately understand the subtle differences between cultural groups. In most cases, however, some sensitivity and awareness makes all the difference.

Case Study: Cultural Misunderstandings.

Simple problems can often arise from cultural misunderstandings. The case study below illustrates this very clearly!

Suleman Pervez moved to the United States from his native Pakistan in the 1950s. With a doctorate in plant pathology and a young family, he had become frustrated with the impossibility of finding well-paid work in his homeland, a developing country. In American, he worked initially as a taxi-driver, and eventually secured a university job. Now, in his eighties, he lives in Ashburn nursing home, restricted by his physical frailty and increasing problems with memory loss and confusion. Two of Mr. Pervez's daughters have returned to Pakistan, where they are married with children of their own, and his son, who lives nearby and manages a large vineyard, felt unable to care for his father properly.

Friends and family have always respected Mr. Pervez's gentleness and compassion, so his son was surprised to be called into the nursing home for a meeting about his father's difficulty in getting along with nursing staff. Early that day, Mr. Pervez had angrily refused his lunch, and had thrown his tray onto the floor, upsetting a bowl of soup which landed on the nurses' aide, scalding her leg quite badly. When he was restrained, he become increasingly angry and disturbed, and the registered nurse on charge had to tranquilize him.

"This is not the first time it's happened," the director of nurses informed Mr. Pervez's son, who is also called Suleman, "and unless there's some improvement in his behavior, he is simply going to have to leave."

It did not take long for Suleman junior to work out the problem. His father is from a Muslim background and although he is not especially devout – he does not observe the frequent prayers that orthodox Muslims are obliged to offer – he has always been careful to avoid eating those foodstuffs that are prohibited by Islam. Already somewhat confused and angry as a result of his deteriorating mental condition, Mr. Pervez was horrified to be given bacon and ham to eat –

not once, but on repeated occasions. What the nurses' aide thought was simply awkward, uncooperative behavior was the patient's observance of the religious code that is central to his cultural background. When Mr. Pervez moved to live in Ashburn nursing home, his son explained his dietary needs, but these were not conveyed to the new nurses' aide, and the kitchen staff were not over concerned with following them. With greater attention to the details of cultural difference, Mr. Pervez's distress, and the injury to the nurses' aide could both have easily been avoided.

Racial Discrimination Towards Healthcare Workers

Healthcare workers are at least as likely as anyone else to suffer from racial discrimination, and, unfortunately, there have been many cases of discrimination within the nursing home environment. While it's hard to deal with the patient with Alzheimer's who has forgotten most things, but remembers his or her dislike of people of another color, there have also been many cases of blatant discrimination on the part of people who should know better. Below, I quote a recent report from the US Equal Employment Opportunity Commission.[38].

EEOC Settles Racial Harassment Suit With St. Louis Nursing Home For $1.2 Million

ST. LOUIS – At a press conference today, the U.S. Equal Employment Opportunity Commission (EEOC) announced a settlement of almost $1.2 million for nine individuals in a racial harassment lawsuit against Beverly Enterprises, Inc., which operates several nursing homes in the St. Louis area. The settlement, which still requires approval of the federal district court here, also requires substantial injunctive relief, including training, monitoring, and disciplinary action against a Beverly human resources employee.

EEOC Chairwoman Ida Castro hailed the resolution: "This case emphasizes that employers cannot condone racially repugnant conduct by their managers or retaliation against those employees who complain. The EEOC's National En-

---

[38] US Equal Employment Opportunity Commission, July 2, 2001.

forcement Plan has targeted such cases involving egregious racial discrimination and we will continue to pursue them vigorously."

In September 1998, the EEOC filed suit under Title VII of the Civil Rights Act of 1964 on behalf of nine former employees alleging racial harassment, retaliation, and unlawful discharge. The suit claimed that the administrator of Beverly's Bridgeton Nursing Center pursued a campaign of flagrant racial harassment against the facility's predominantly black workforce during 1993 and 1994. She frequently used racial slurs to refer to black employees and ordered white supervisors and charge nurses to discipline black employees without cause. The administrator also required applications to be coded with smiling faces for white applicants and frowning faces for black applicants. When some black and white employees refused to follow or complained about her discriminatory practices, she retaliated by discharging them or forcing them to resign.

Discrimination towards healthcare workers who are also members of ethnic minorities can also come from the people that they are hired to care for – the residents, and sometimes also their families. All nursing home residents are vulnerable, by definition. Mostly elderly, they suffer from a range of health problems, and are often confused or even demented. None of this, however, excludes the possibility that they may also be profoundly racist, and resent finding themselves in the care of someone whom they perceive to be inferior. To be blunt, a person who is old and vulnerable is not necessarily a pleasant, gentle person. One who has been a bigoted racist in youth will not cease to be so simply because of age. With the onset of Alzheimer's disease comes a lowering of inhibitions, and it is not infrequent for sufferers of Alzheimer's to use offensive racial terms of the sort that I would rather not reproduce here, and even to resort to physical violence against their carer. What can be done? Truthfully, very little. Someone in the grips of Alzheimer's disease is not a person to be reasoned with. As distasteful as it is, nurses' aides, nurses and other healthcare workers have to tolerate appalling abuse at times. A salient issue here is one of payment. Nurses' aides especially are, as we have already established, among the worst paid workers in the United States. Their work is difficult, arduous, riddled with work-related ailments and repetitive strain injuries. And as if that were not bad enough, nurses' aides are also often subjected to torrents of racial abuse. They endure a lot, for very little financial reward.

Another appalling aspect of being a member of a racial or ethnic minority employed in nursing home are the reactions of racist family members. Angered by real or perceived discrepancies in the care received by their elderly parents (problems which are generally caused by the usual issues of understaffing and underfunding), some family members lash out and blame nurses' aides, accusing them of misconduct, and attributing this to their racial or ethnic background. It is hard for the typical nurses' aide, thus attacked, to find retribution. Racist slurs in the nursing home environment are just one more reason for the high turnover of burned-out, underpaid nurses' aides who leave the profession every year.

Racism towards Nursing Home Residents

As we mentioned above, some discrepancies in the care of residents can be attributed to thoughtlessness and a lack of cultural sensitivity rather than to blatant racism. Cultural insensitivity can be fought by educating healthcare workers, and often simply by gently reminding them to be aware of cultural difference. Blatant racism towards nursing home residents is another matter. It may not be common, but one incident is one incident too many.

Portrait of a Culturally Integrated Nursing Home

When Bayview Heights changed ownership five years ago, the new administrator, Steven Harris, realized that he would have his work cut out. In a racially and ethnically mixed neighborhood, the home catered to elders from a variety of backgrounds – White, African American, Mexican and more. Although there were only 65 residents, those still well enough to take part in activities tended to stay with people from their own background, and each group seemed to view the other with a degree of suspicion. Then, of course, as in so many nursing homes, the nurses' aides were mostly young women who had recently emigrated to the United States from nations as diverse as the Philippines and Ethiopia. Families of residents didn't always help, either. In most respects the home was well run and organized, but the tensions among both residents and staff caused a living environment that could be difficult at times. Steven could see that this was not due – in the case of the vast majority of residents, families and nursing staff – to racism, but to a lack of familiarity with different cultures. The remedy was easier than anyone could have imagined. Bayview Heights added to its list of activities the celebration of the various national holidays. On the 5th of May, the Mexican national holiday, the kitchen prepared Latin American dishes, and the Mexican-American residents were encouraged to sing their traditional songs. On another occasion, two of the nurses' aides, from the Philippines, were asked to give a presentation about their country and culture. An Ethiopian nurse brought in samples of clothing and jewelry made in her town. With the lively ethnic mix, it wasn't hard to arrange events. Residents' families were invited to these presentations, which served to break down barriers. Although a few residents remained reluctant to mix with others, most were happy to recognize that they shared much more with the others than they had ever expected. While the usual problems of under-staffing and under-funding have not gone away, Bayview has a much more relaxed atmosphere than before. Even the kitchen staff, who originally grumbled when they were asked to prepare ethnic foods, now enjoy the change which has become a fortnightly ritual. Attendance of activities has increased considerably, and more of the residents are spending time in the living and social areas rather than in their rooms. Achieving this level of cultural integration is considered by Steven to be his greatest success as an administrator, and he tries to focus on it when the difficulty of keeping the home afloat seems too much to cope with.

The cultural diversity that prevails in the United States is one of the things that makes it a fascinating, and ethnically rich nation. Dealing with ethnic difference can be challenging – and all the more so in the context of a nursing home. But the problems that cultural differences can raise are not insurmountable, and the rewards of learning how to manage them are worth the effort.

CHAPTER TEN: BEING THE BOSS

When I began working as a nursing home administrator, I spent some time with each resident everyday, even if I only had enough time to say hello. During my many years in the business, I have met a long of wonderful people from every walk of life – teachers, attorneys, housewives, painters, war heroes, railroad workers ... none are less than full human beings, regardless of the extent of their incapacity. Often, we developed a warm relationship, and it has been overwhelming to have to see them grow weak with age. On the other hand, it is heart-warming to see families, residents and staff to work together to create the best possible way of meeting the residents' needs. Over the years, I found the process of befriending residents, only to lose them when their lives came to a close, increasingly stressful. The ability of nurses to spend their professional lives doing this never ceases to amaze and impress me. I could never have been a therapist!

Upgrades and Improvements

As a caregiver, administrator, inspector and owner of nursing homes, my priority has always been to struggle to provide the best possible environment for the elderly for whom I am responsible. I first began to understand the huge negative effect of understaffing when I worked as an inspector, and I have always striven to persuade management and owners to increase staffing levels, although they often had to increase their budgets to become able to do so. I felt strongly about the issue as perhaps the most significant deficiency I saw in nursing homes was understaffing. Nurses simply did not have time to complete their assignments. Staffing levels were based upon the budget of the home and not on the level of care needed. Nothing has changed, and nor has the response of nursing home owners when they are challenged about their staffing levels: "How can we increase it when the government will not increase our daily rate?"

When I became a nursing home owner, the first task I put into action was to increase our staffing ration of one nurses' aide to every ten patients, to one to every six. We also hired more licensed nurses to supervise aides and provide qualified nursing care. With these increases in staffing, the quality of life of the residents improved enormously, and we still have one of the best staffed facilities in the Bay Area. I would still like to see higher staffing levels, but this is not possible, even though we have started to offer subacute care, a type of care that brings with it more intense staffing levels. There just are not enough nurses to fill all the necessary positions to care for residents properly.

Changes in Medicare policy affected us in 1983, when the government decided to change the way it paid for Medicare patients in acute hospitals, implementing a diagnosis related system of payment – a fixed rate reimbursement system, with a fixed number of days in hospital. Hospital budgets collapsed under the strain of the new system, and administrators were forced to cut costs. One way in which they did so was by discharging Medicare patients more quickly, resulting in seriously ill people being transferred to nursing homes or to their own homes. In response to this situation, some nursing homes – including ours – became equipped to provide subacute care. We began to admit patients with graver health problems, and more complex medical issues. The cost of care increased, and so did revenue, and we expanded our facilities and increased our staffing numbers. Our goal was to provide top quality care and treatment for patients using ventilators, or with other complicated health needs. To help us to do this, we hired some excellent nursing staff, many of whom are still working with us today. As well as adding to our nursing staff, we took on professional social workers, dietitians and support personnel including a subacute director. To maintain a high standard of medical care we contracted with a physician to be on duty for forty hours a week. We also upgraded our facilities, by purchasing inline oxygen systems and suctioning systems for patients on ventilators. Payments from insurance companies and Medicare increased – Medicare payment did not fully support the cost of care, and had to be supplemented with private and insurance payment.

Success Stories

Working in a nursing home can be tough. Many, if not most, nursing home residents will not leave until they die. Helping people to live as well as possible and die with dignity is one of the most important functions of a nursing home. Running a sub-acute facility for medically complex patients, however, does provide one with the opportunity to help people to live full lives again, returning to their homes and embracing many of their favorite activities. Let me introduce you to some of the patients and former patients of our facility.

Steve

Steve was admitted to our facility with severe traumatic brain injury in 1995, following a fall. He had a subarachnoid hemorrhage and non depressed parietial/ocipital skull fracture, and presented with severe spastic quadriparesis. On evaluation, he was seen to have a very limited range of motion, cervical right side bending and rotation left knee 90 degree flexion contracture. Our physician-led team developed a plan which included serial casting to left knee to restore extension, truck and neck balancing exercises, passive stretching exercises to left leg, splinting lower extremities, bed mobility training, transfer training, walking activities utilizing a tilt table, family education and therapeutic exercises to lower extremities. All of this resulted in an increase in mobility. At the beginning, Steve needed a lot of assistance to perform even the simplest task, but soon he was able to do a lot by himself with verbal prompting. He went from depending on two assistants to do everything to requiring only one from time to time. He became able to sit and stand on his own and hold his head upright.

Ongoing physical therapy yielded remarkable progress. When he was admitted, Steve was only able to use simple words, and became extremely upset when he failed to understand verbal commands. Soon he was able to follow instructions to perform tasks such as grooming and hygiene. His attention span increased from nil, to remaining alert for up to 45 minutes, and responding in an appropriate fashion to verbal cues. Socially, his response to external stimuli and family members increased. His auditory, visual and sensory functioning also increased significantly.

Steve's success can be attributed to the dedicated persistence of experienced staff, who constantly evaluated and adjusted therapy, and to the planned involvement of family and friends throughout the process. In the nursing facility, we were very proud to receive a recommendation letter from the attending physician of the referring hospital.

Gloria

Gloria was admitted to the facility with a rare condition – botulism-type paralysis, which left her in a quadriplegic condition, suffering from double vision, dysphagia and dysathria and difficulty clearing secretions. She also had a history of depression. Prior to entering the subacute facility, she was treated in hospital, where her condition deteriorated to the extent that she needed ventilator assistance for breathing.

Upon transfer to our facility, our team of therapists and pulmonary, neurological and psychiatric physician consultants worked closely together with our in-house physician, Gloria, and her family. Every small improvement was a triumph for us all, and we became close in the process of helping Gloria to recover. She improved gradually, from being a total quadriplegic in need of a ventilator, to being able to produce weak shoulder shrugs and movement of neck, shoulders and right arm. Gloria was fitted with a customized laser pointer and alpha board to improve her communication. She resumed speech after a Passy Muir Valve was implemented. Her mental condition also improved, and her fears receded to the point whereby she was able to transfer to the state of Washington to be cared for by her family.

Mary

Mary, aged 70, was admitted with a diagnosis of post fracture Left Proximal fibular and multi-system diseases (ASHD, CHF, Diabetes Mellitus, Chronic Venous Insufficiency). She was also grossly obese, weighing more than 300 pounds. She had already lived in several nursing homes, and had not walked for two years.

Our interdisciplinary approach, which included intensive psychological encouragement, prompted great improvement. Mary's functional ability increased enormously. Initially, she needed help with everything, but she progressed to using a front wheel walker which she used to take her from bed to chair, and then to a walker which she uses to walk distances of up to 100 feet. With pain management and psychological support, Mary has been able to transcend the emotional and pain barriers and achieve success. She has also lost over 50 pounds, and plans to go home soon.

Susan

Susan, who is 95 years old, was admitted to our facility with multiple diagnoses. It was no longer possible for her daughter to take care of her at home. Initially, Susan found it extremely difficult to adjust to the routine of the facility, so the recreational therapist started a one to one coping and adjustment program. With twice daily visits using therapeutic counseling, Susan became more comfortable with her new surroundings. Although she initially refused to join in any of the activities on offer, she eventually began to attend. She particularly enjoyed the therapeutic movement class, because she was able to do all the movements. Although she'd never played bingo before, she decided to try the game – and now she loves it! She marks her own card and often wins. Together with her daughter, she has participated in various social events and feels generally good about living in the nursing facility.

Curt

Curt, a 62 year old man, entered the facility with diagnoses of respiratory failure, aspiration pneumonia, colic disease, psychiatric disorders and a history of acute abdomen pain with small intestinal perforation. He was fed with a PEG tube, because he had difficulty swallowing and weight loss as well as chronic diarrhea. In layman's terms, Curt was wasting away. Our registered dietician assessed Curt on admission and ordered a gluten-free diet. After a few days, the diarrhea cleared, and it has not returned. Nurses and speech therapists worked with Curt in developing proper eating procedures so that he could eat slowly and prevent aspiration. Curt is now having his meals in the dining room, tolerating his special meals well, and gaining weight – about nine pounds in one month. Tube feeding is no longer necessary. Curt feels that he is in control of his body, will probably be reducing his anti-depressant drugs and is making plans to go back home.

Consuela

Consuela has earned the respect and praise of all of our staff and residents for her determination to improve her situation. She was admitted to our facility with a speech and voice disorder, dysarthria and dysphonia. She was also suffering from dysphagia and an open wound from graft sites on her left thigh. She was considerably underweight on admission – just 100 pounds, when she stands 5'2". After following an intense course with our speech therapist, she learned how to speak clearly and audibly. She now eats all of her meals and has gained seven pounds in weight. Her wounds have begun to heal. Soon, Consuela will be able to go home, or at least to an alternative board and care facility.

The opportunity I've had to play a part in providing good subacute care at my nursing facility has been one of my greatest sources of pride in recent years, and I do feel that the incorporation of subacute facilities into nursing homes has vast potential. But will the funding bodies allow this potential to flourish?

CHAPTER ELEVEN: ONWARD AND UPWARD

We are fast reaching a state of tolerance for the deplorable conditions in our nursing homes, as we grow hardened to the current reality of abuse and neglect and nursing care to minimal standards of acceptability. Nursing home administrators and owners have become resigned to a reality in which it is no longer possible to provide adequate care to elderly residents. Numbed by the impossibility of the situation, many residents' families are reaching the same unhappy state of resignation. But we must not allow ourselves to start thinking that quality care and a happy, homelike environment are unattainable for our senior citizens. We *can* work together to make things better, and if we do, the rewards of our labors will start to be seen before long.

Currently, the federal and state governments' answer to inadequate care is to issue erring nursing homes with citations and fines, rather than to provide proactive solutions towards improving service. So long as this continues, nursing homes will become used to paying fines, and will consider them to be an inevitable cost of conducting business, as unimportant as traffic tickets. But nothing will change. Until we *decide* that things must improve and start taking steps to make them do so, the elderly will still be left in nursing homes, confined to beds in institutions that allow 80 square feet per person. Their care will be documented and assessed and evaluated to show – to the inspectors' satisfaction if not that of the residents themselves – that basic needs such as food, a clean bed and room, an activity program and basic activities are being catered for. As long as the documentation shows that a decline in residents' health is due to natural and not administrative problems, inspectors will ask no questions. Nurses will continue to be overworked, work related injuries will continue to occur and insurance rates will continue to rise.

Under these conditions, it will become more and more difficult for small nursing homes to cope, and these will, with a dreary inevitability, be consolidated into chains whose business it is to generate profits, not to maximize the quality of care. Old people in need of help will have become no more than any other commodity.

The Crisis in America's Nursing Homes

When nursing homes are owned by public corporations whose intention it is to generate profits, individuals cannot be blamed for the abuse or neglect of elderly residents. Corporations can shoulder the burden of the fines that will inevitably be issued and there will be little incentive to improve the quality of care. Jobs may be terminated, but it will be easy for abusive staff to move to another nursing home, and mete out the same treatment to another vulnerable patient. As so many nursing home employees are taken on at entry level, with no prior training in the field, abusive staff can always find employment. Corporate directors and CEOs are never held responsible when these atrocities occur. When fines are issued, the corporation shoulders the debt, not management. So long as homes are run as businesses, the bottom line will always be profit and not resident welfare. On the other hand, homes owned by single individuals are easy targets when the government wants to lash out and make an example of someone. A private owner does not have the financial clout of a large corporation, and, quite simply, cannot fight against the might of the government of the United States.

If we want to break this circle of abuse, we must do so now. If we believe that our senior citizens are valued members of society, we must make this known. If we want to be confident that we will be cared for in our own old age, we must start to implement reforms. Our retirement funds will not protect us from ill health and the need for nursing home care and services.

But where should we begin? We need to begin by taking a long, hard look at the current system of price control and the manner in which regulations are enforced by issuing fines and citations. By placing the emphasis on cost and on punishments that affect homes financially, we are stressing the wrong criteria. Reducing the issue of the care of the elderly to dollars and cents shifts the focus of healthcare from the patients onto the budget and overheads, and treatment from what's best for the patient to a set of prescribed protocols. Suffering from disease X? You need treatment Y! This is how much it costs ... Meals become examples of economy and activities time-slots that must be filled to keep inspectors happy.

If this system continues, we will raise a generation of Americans that, quite simply, knows no other way. It will come to believe that this type of care is inevitable. Those who complain to City Hall will learn that this is just the way that things are done. The situation will only change if demands are made to state and federal government. Families will have to set aside the problems of everyday life – work, children and leisure hours – to make their representation to government. The abuse of individual elders is currently addressed in small-scale lawsuits and civil actions. Individual families complain. Some will see their complaints addressed, but many will not. But the abuse of one nursing home resident diminishes us all. The neglect of any Medicare recipient should be a source of shame to the public in general.

Never forget that the taxpayer funds Medicare and Medicaid. Taxpayers – in short, you and I – must insist that we get good value for our investment!

As you can see, compassion, love and understanding for the nature of human beings are totally lacking in the care and treatment of our elderly sick and disabled. Nursing homes and the government between them have generated a level of care resulting in a situation whereby our elderly live the remainder of their lives in barely acceptable conditions. The basic requisites are that residents be free from infliction of physical pain or injury; chemical or physical control beyond the physician's order; the infliction of mental or emotional suffering; disregard for the necessities of daily living; lack of care for existing medical problems; creating situations harmful to the resident's self-esteem; illegal or improper use of a resident's property for personal gain.

Too many nursing homes provide care that would not even be acceptable in a zoo. Why? Not because the nursing staff are cruel individuals, but because their workloads do not permit them to give the quality of care their dependants need. The organization of nursing homes, and the federal government's price control only covers minimum costs. We are forced to accept the lowest possible standard of care for our elderly and to create a work environment unappealing to those who would become nursing professionals if they could see a way to realize their professional aspirations within the industry.

Towards a Better Future

How can we ensure that the nursing homes of the future are better, not worse, than they are today? The first step we need to take is to make a mental shift from the acceptance of inadequate care for our senior citizens to demanding more, and looking for realistic solutions to the problem. We have already identified the key problems extant in nursing home care today: insufficient federal funding; inadequate staffing levels; poor remuneration for healthcare workers; unpleasant working environments; cumbersome regulations and the homogenization of healthcare as the private sector scrabbles for profits. How can these issues be addressed? Currently, America stands convicted of indifference. Now, for just a moment, let's imagine that we live in a country truly committed to providing high quality healthcare to its senior citizens. Let's suppose that our nation's elders are a high priority to our politicians. Let's completely lose our grasp on reality and envision an America that genuinely wants to do the best it can for its oldest, most vulnerable inhabitants. In such a dream-world, what solutions are presented? How can elderly people in need of care be catered for with dignity and respect? What sort of a system will use taxpayers' hard-earned contributions effectively, and get the money to where it's needed? Is such a system even feasible?

One change in strategy that would help would be to develop senior healthcare living centers, by purchasing land for nursing homes in rural areas or outside major cities where it is less costly, thus freeing more money to care for residents. If healthcare centers were located in large complexes – perhaps incorporating several institutions beneath a single roof – construction costs per room would be lower, and a wider range of specialized staff would be able to work on the premises, providing a complete healthcare service without need of hiring in experts on a costly consultative basis. Rural settings would provide more outdoor space for recreational activities, and allow for the construction of larger indoor facilities. Careful selection of locations would allow homes to cater for families living in various different urban centers at the same time. Different ethnic-religious groups could be catered for by centralizing most services but, for example, having various dining areas offering kosher, halal and other specialized diets as necessary.

Is there more that could be done? There certainly is! In this ideal world, the government does not nurse the fear that socialized medicine will introduce the specter of left-wing political and economic stratagems, threatening the American Way of free enterprise. The federalization of nursing homes would eliminate profit as a reason for providing substandard nursing home care. It would also ensure that facilities were built and catered to by subsidized government contracts. Standards of care would become consistently higher around the country, with centralized departments and services monitoring and providing services. Higher qualifications would become necessary for those applying to work in nursing homes, with a corresponding increase in salaries and professional expectations. Above all, an audit policy that is proactive rather than disciplinary would be devised. In other words, deficiencies would be treated as opportunities to work for improvement rather than occasions to punish institutions by issuing financial penalties. Federalization would also eliminate the need for an inspection and enforcement program, as federal employees would now be in charge of nursing care, and would have no driving force other than that of providing a high quality of care. The government, now directly responsible for the standard of living of the elders of America, would no longer be able to blame private corporations for problems, and would have to take responsibility.

This might sound like an impossible dream, but it really isn't. The federal government already has a long history of managing hospitals and nursing homes for the nation's veterans. The basic model of a centralized healthcare system is already in place: the nursing homes and other healthcare facilities run by the Veteran Administration. Veterans' homes may not be perfect, but they definitely represent a big step in the right direction. Since as long ago as 1811, the Veteran Administration has delivered continuous healthcare services, when federal government authorized the first medical facility for veterans. The civil war prompted the establishment of many more such facilities on both sides of the struggle, and in the years that followed, poor and disabled veterans from the Indian and Spanish-American wars and from the Mexican border were all cared for in these institutions. America's entry into the fray that was the First World War prompted Congress and the American public to recognize the need to establish a system of healthcare benefits for veterans. The Veterans' Administration in its current form was founded in 1930, and today it manages 171 medical centers as well as more than 130 outpatient, community and outreach clinics, 126 nursing home units and 35 domiciliary units, which between them offer a wide variety of medical, surgical and rehabilitative care. In 1989, President Bush established a cabinet level position for the Administration, saying, "There is only one place for the veterans of America – in the Cabinet Room, at the table with the President of the United States of America."

Veterans have given all they have to fight for their country, but they are not the only ones whose struggles built the America we live in today. What about veterans' widows? What about the men and women who have developed agriculture, industry, science and education? The mothers who struggled to balance work and family? The parents who worked tirelessly to ensure that their children would be able to get an education? All of these people, in one way or another, have helped to build America. In their declining years, their contribution should be applauded, and rewarded by providing them with a decent standard of living. Isn't the best place for our seniors in the Cabinet Room, at table with the President of the United States of America?

As a people, we should make it our mission to serve Medicare and Medicaid residents and their families with compassion and respect. We should recognize their contribution to the growth of our nation by ensuring that they receive the care they need in old age, and that it is given with dignity. This should be our vision for the new millennium.

CHAPTER TWELVE: MAKING THE BEST OF IT

If you've reached that difficult moment when you're forced to recognize that your aged mother or father needs more help than can be provided, you need to be sure that you choose the best possible option available. As I think I've made abundantly clear, nursing home care in American today is far from ideal – but there are ways of making the service you receive as good as it can possibly be. So, take a few days off work if necessary, don't let anyone bully or hassle you to make a rushed decision and invest some time in your future peace of mind, and in the comfort and happiness of someone you love.

Nursing Home Information in the Public Domain

Many state authorities, and the Medicare program, have published information on how to choose a nursing home. Usually, this information is available both in printed form and on the Internet. It generally takes the form of a check-list of regulation requirements. If you use the Internet, check the web-pages of your state authority for the basic information – names of nursing homes, their locations and the services they provide. Some federal and state agencies provide details of the latest inspection reports on the Medicare website, `<http://www.medicare.gov>`. Typing "nursing home" or "nursing home care" into any search engine will bring up a host of information sites for you to look at. Much of the information may be useful, but, as always, treat unofficial sites on the Internet with caution.

Make your Own Decision

When a family member is ill and in hospital, it is easy to let important decisions be taken from one's hands. Often, hospitals tell family members that they are arranging the discharge of a patient to a certain nursing home because a vacancy has arisen, and that the patient has to leave because Medicare payments have ceased. At this stage, many hospitals push families into accepting decisions quickly, and there is often little or no time for visits to the nursing home before accepting their services. At stressful moments, it's all too easy to let someone take responsibility out of one's hands. The most frequent scenario is for the hospital discharge planner to supply a list of nursing homes in the area, and send you off to look, or to simply inform you that your elderly mother or father is being transferred to a particular facility in a couple of days. Don't let yourself be pushed around! *You have the right to refuse discharge from an acute hospital until you have found a nursing home that is acceptable to you* – and don't let the hospital authorities forget it. The nursing home business is an industry, it's true – a *service* industry. The resident, their family, and/or the government is buying that service and, as with everything that is paid for, should find out what will be given in exchange for their money. Would you buy the first car you were offered, or purchase an expensive outfit without seeing it? No. And this is immeasurably more important. Take time to get prepared and choose the right nursing home, one that employs sufficient staff, and is run by an administrator and director of nurses whom you feel you can trust. Don't assume that the hospital's discharge planner is an impartial judge of nursing facilities. Hospitals and nursing homes have close business relationships, and may have come to mutually beneficial financial agreements. The discharge owner might be a personal friend or associate of the administrator or director of nurses of a particular home. How much more families should do when finding a home for our elderly family members! It does take a lot of work to find the right nursing home, but this is an investment, not only in the future well being of the resident, but in your own peace of mind. If you are confident that you have explored the options and chosen the most viable one, you will be able to leave your mother or father in their new home without torturing yourself with doubts and self-criticism.

Choosing

How to choose? Well, even once you've done the initial donkey work of short-listing all the possibly suitable homes in your area, there is still a lot to do. Have you found a nursing home that looks promising? Take your time to be sure, and visit more than once. Find opportunities to talk to the administrator, director of nurses, food service supervisor, activity leader and other key staff members, and try to get to know them as individuals as well as healthcare providers. Of course, your main topics of conversation will be about the services they provide, but talk about items of general interest too, and develop a friendly rapport. Use your common sense and keep your eyes open to see if the residents are offered activities, and whether or not there seems to be a healthy, respectful relationship between residents and staff. If your family member needs special care, such as physical therapy or psychiatric treatment, talk to the relevant professionals, and ensure that these services will be available and that they have a full understanding of their needs. Do you still feel positive about the home after several visits? Before finalizing your decision, ask the administrator or director of nurses about the most recent inspection report. These are public information, and a copy should be posted in an area where anyone has access to it. The nursing home is obliged to give you a copy if you ask for one. Bear in mind that the inspections, which are conducted every nine to fifteen months, are there to highlight deficiencies, and issue fines and other penalties and not to talk about the positive aspects of the care provided by the facility. Nursing homes are required to respond to the deficiencies listed in the report, and you may also ask to read these responses. If a nursing home refuses to supply you with an inspection report, or tries to distract you from asking for it, there may well be a good reason. You are entitled to insist. Never overlook the valuable information that can often be found close to home by asking friends, relatives and community workers such as local clergy, doctors and attorneys. If you can, try to get in touch with the families of people already cared for in the nursing home you're looking at, and ask if they're reasonably happy with the service provided. Back up information you get informally by checking with federal and state programs that assist seniors from the Office on Aging and the long-term care ombudsman in your area. These government agencies are not allowed to favor one home over another, but must provide impartial data in the form of inspection reports.

Above all, never forget that, no matter how much research you do, you should always visit and get to know an institution for yourself. Below, you'll find comprehensive checklists to help you make the right decision.

Work with the Home

Choosing the right nursing home for your mother or father is a daunting task, and the work doesn't stop there. Once your family member is installed, you can choose between working with the home to make their new life as comfortable and rewarding as possible, or being passive, and leaving the nurses and other caregivers with sole responsibility. If you decide to be passive, you will be partly responsible if your parent or aged relative is unhappy. Nurses and nurses' aides are healthcare professionals, not psychics. They don't know residents' likes and dislikes straight away. As ever, it takes time to build a relationship. You can help make that relationship a healthy one, by proposing alternatives instead of criticizing, by joining in group and family activities and by working with staff to encourage everything that is positive about the care they offer. All nursing homes are imperfect – choose the best option available, and then contribute to making it better. In some ways, having an elderly parent in a nursing home is like having a child in school. Take an interest in their activities and interests, while bearing in mind that they have changed, and may no longer be able to do the same things that they did when they were younger. Your parents adapted to you when you were a child, and now the roles have reversed. If one of the nursing home staff makes an honest slip of judgment, try to say something like: " I think you'll find my mother more cooperative if you give her more time to get dressed," instead of: "Why did you make her rush so much? Can't you see that that was the wrong thing to do?"

Don't let things slide when your mother or father has settled in. Visit the nursing home as often as you can. If, for whatever reason, you are unable to visit every day or every week, get in touch with friends or relatives living nearby and ask them to drop in as often as they can so that you can call them for a progress report. Keep in touch with the nursing home staff by telephone, even if only for a few minutes every day. Your calls will keep them aware of your concern, and they will respond to it. You probably try to enjoy a friendly professional relationship with your doctor, your dentist and the staff in your local video outlet – how much more important it is to be able to speak amicably with your parent's care providers!

Settling In

Be realistic, and don't expect your mother or father to be immediately happy in their nursing home. It's important to understand that it takes some time to settle in, and adjust to change. Before they move, sit down with them and talk through their doubts and worries, assuring them that you will always be there for them. If the home you've chosen is a good one, the staff will do all they can to help residents feel comfortable in their new surroundings – but moving house is always stressful, and this doesn't change with age. Even if the resident in question is confused and unsure of his or her whereabouts, the strange new location will take some getting used to. Make things as easy as possible by asking staff to provide familiar meals at customary times, and by bringing in personal items such as photographs and favorite ornaments. If pets are being left behind, ensure that they are given new homes, and that progress reports about their welfare will be available. Find out if they can come to visit, too. Send out change of address notification to any of your parent's correspondents. Little touches like putting together a family album with photographs recording happy events in the past will help.

Alternatives to Nursing Home Care

What if your aged family member is no longer able to live alone, but not in need of full nursing home care? There are a number of possibilities available. If your family can afford it, it may be possible to hire someone to come and stay in the home to care for them. Costs are high, however, running to twice that of nursing home care. Community resources including meals on wheels and other adult day care services may also be available. Alternately, assisted living is possible. Seniors who live in this environment are provided with their own housing unit comprising a small apartment with a bedroom and bathroom. They can avail of central dining services, laundry services, and limited housekeeping, or make arrangements privately. The resident pays a monthly rent, with extra fees for other services. Another option is a board and care home. These small group homes cater for residents who do not need nursing services, but benefit from assistance with eating, walking, bathing and visiting the toilet. Assess your parent's needs carefully

– if nursing home care is not essential, there may be a better answer to your situation.

The Rights of the Individual

Every nursing home is obliged to provide its residents with the care and services they need to reach their highest possible level of physical, mental and social well being –even though only a minority has succeeded in providing this fully. The state and federal governments pass law after law, but only nursing home staff can provide the care and services necessary to making the residents' lives as pleasant as possible – and regardless of how well-meaning and caring the staff is, they can only work with the tools and expertise they've got. Government laws only guarantee minimal services, as the standard of quality and care considered necessary has been lowered to unacceptable levels. Unless you do your research carefully, you can only depend upon a bed, three meals a day, a bath once a week and a monthly 5 minute consultation with a physician. Do the best you can to find the right nursing home for your parent, but don't let unrealistic expectations set you up for disappointment.

We are all unique – and this applies as much to the elderly as to anybody else. Nursing staff should be aware of each resident's personal likes and dislikes so that they can accommodate at least some of them. The basic human needs for respect, encouragement, friendship and autonomy should never be forgotten. The fact that they often *are* is reflected in the depression that is widespread among the elderly, who see their deaths approaching as they lose control over their own daily activities. Many become institutionalized rapidly, learning to accept that the staff will make every decision for them. The inability of many nursing homes to allow reasonable degrees of autonomy is directly related to understaffing and underfunding. Freedom and privacy are sacrificed to rules and schedules.

The best way to secure as many basic, individual rights for your mother or father is to become involved in their care plan, and to encourage them to be as proactive as they can be. While they are settling in to their new home, you should try to be present at mealtimes, to talk to the activity director and to the nursing staff in charge of their care, and to oversee their washing and dressing, until they feel more comfortable with their new surroundings.

Be Aware of Nursing Home Abuse and Neglect

Major concerns in nursing homes today are the use of chemical and physical restraints, inadequate supply of foods or fluids and other forms of abuse and neglect. In order to protect residents from the overuse of restraints, and more, they have been given many rights under state and federal law. Ideally, these rights should prevent the nursing home from taking advantage of the resident. Sadly, this is not always the case. It is your responsibility to review these rights and understand them. If your elderly parent is restrained, either physically or chemically, find out why. Has the restraint been ordered by a physician? Many families worry that nursing home physicians will order restraints for the convenience of the nursing staff rather than the welfare of the resident – do everything you can to ensure that unnecessary restraints are not ordered. If you have doubts about the performance of any nursing home member of staff, don't hesitate to ask about his or her background. Was a criminal check run before they were hired? Have there been complaints about them before? Regular visiting is important to ensure that your parent is not mistreated in any way. Check their legs and arms for unexplained bruises and make sure that they are kept clean. Sudden weight loss should always be asked about.

Religious, Cultural, and Language Preferences

It is important that nursing home residents be as happy as they can be. Crucial to their wellbeing is that they feel comfortable in their surroundings. If your elderly relative has specific religious, linguistic or cultural needs, try to find a home that will accommodate them. Jews, Muslims and Hindus, for example, need to be confident that they will be provided with meals acceptable to their faith's dietary laws. Roman Catholics need to know that they will be able to receive communion on Sundays, and confess when they feel the need. Spanish speakers should be able to communicate with at least some staff members. Similarly, if your primary language is English, be sure that staff members and residents can understand and speak it. Ensure that religious leaders – be they priests, rabbis or whatever – can come and visit as required. If religious images or other furnishings are important to your family, make sure that they can be brought into the home. If your parent is religious, the presence of a sacred image on his or her bedside will be a comfort. Try to arrange to have a religious leader pay a visit shortly after moving in, and ask him or her to assure availability in case of crisis. Most ethnic groups have their own recipes and types of food. While you can't expect the kitchen staff to be experts in international cuisine, you can try to visit with snacks or meals that will remind your relative of home.

Resolving Problems

Problems may arise from time to time, even in the best nursing home. The extent to which these will affect the resident in question depends largely on the reaction of the family. When difficulties arise, the first thing you should ask is whether or not the nursing home has enough staff. Understaffing is the number one cause of problems, from inefficiency to abuse. Do you feel confident in approaching the authorities in the home to discuss the issue? – you should! When you discuss problems, be careful not to paint yourself as a troublemaker or a threat to the staff. Rather than calling the state authorities to complain the moment something goes wrong, try to work with nurses, aides and administration to fix it. Calling in government authorities results in citations and fines, but rarely in a concrete improvement in conditions. Even worse, if you and your family are seen as difficult, this may have serious repercussions for your elderly relative, who may become subject to abuse or neglect on the part of angry staff members. Before resorting to government officials – which is, sadly, necessary from time to time – talk the issue through with the nursing home manager. Most want to work with you, and deal with your concerns. Only when friendly attempts to resolve the problem have failed should you go to the authorities.

How to Pay

Nursing home care is not cheap. Those who qualify for Medicare will rely on this initially- it pays 100% of care for the first 20 days, following which residents will be expected to pay a co-insurance amount of around $100 a day for the next 80 days. Most residents won't receive more than 20 days of coverage, following which personal assets and savings will have to be used for skilled nursing care to a tune of $150-$200 a day, or more if subacute care is necessary. On entering a nursing home, a contract will be provided for the resident or their family to sign. This will inform you of the basic rates charged for the various services. Basic rates should cover a shared bedroom, meals, housekeeping, linen, general nursing care, recreation and some personal care services. There may be extra charges for personal services, such as haircuts, manicures, television and telephones, and you must take care that there is no confusion about what is charged as extra and what is not.

If the nursing home has a contract with the managed care company you use, a managed care plan may cover some of the cost. Medicare supplemental insurance is private insurance that will pay for any deductible costs and co-insurance that Medicare doesn't cover. The benefits and costs of insurance companies vary widely, but ideally provide a source of funds to ensure that your loved one will receive access to good nursing homes, and fund the services he or she needs. Hopefully, you will have time to research all your payment options without undue haste – even if your mother or father is still well enough to stay at home, it may be wise to do some basic research for the future.

Questions you Should Ask the Nursing Home

Don't let yourself be intimidated by nursing home staff or the situation. Before making your decision, ask about what you can expect. Here are some questions that will help.

- How are roommates chosen? What if my parent and his/her roommate don't get along? Can we request a transfer?
- How are differences resolved between residents and staff?
- Are there any restrictions on visitation?
- How will the home provide the best service it can?
- What kind of interaction is allowed between staff and residents? Are friendships allowed to develop, or are relationships kept on a purely professional level?
- How do you conduct comprehensive assessments?

- Who develops the care plan?
- Can the resident and their family become involved in setting and achieving the treatment goals?
- What protective devices are used, and which are paid for by the government?
- Should we provide skin care ourselves?
- How do you guarantee proper skin nutrition and hydration?
- How do you guarantee a balanced diet?
- Does the home do background checks on its employees for a history of abuse?
- Do the home and its administrator have licenses issued by the state to operate?
- What special services does the home have? Rehabilitation? Subacute/ ventilator care/etc.?
- Does the home have ongoing educational programs for staff to teach them about avoiding abuse, dealing with difficult residents and more?
- How does the home conduct investigations and resolve complaints?
- How does the home safeguard residents' possessions? What happens if something goes missing?
- What activity programs are available?
- What activities are offered outside the facility?
- Do outside volunteers come in?
- Where will the prospective resident's room be?
- How many people stay in each room?
- Are private rooms available?
- Will the room and bed be held if the patient needs to go to hospital?
- Can married couples share a room?
- Can residents add their own items to the room?
- When rooms are shared, are provisions made for privacy, such as curtains around the bed?
- Are the activity personnel trained?

- Are there planned outings?
- Do residents participate in planning activities?
- Can they take part in community activities outside the home?
- Is there a store where they can buy small items?
- Do residents take part in its operation?
- Are extra charges involved in taking part in activities?
- How many lounge areas are available to residents?
- Is there enough room for visitors, conversation, TV watching, etc.?
- Are they clean, comfortably furnished and pleasantly decorated?
- Is there a smoking area where smokers can sit without disturbing others?
- Is there an outside area for residents that is safe and inviting?
- Can residents select their meals from a menu, or select their mealtime?
- If they need help eating, do care plans specify what sort of help they'll receive?
- Can they choose with whom they'll eat?
- How often does the menu change?
- Are fresh fruits and vegetables served?
- Can wine or beer be served, so long as the doctor says it's acceptable?
- Can the resident's family arrange to dine with them in the facility?
- Is it possible to eat in one's room?
- Is consultation with a dietician available?
- Is there a resident council?
- Does it influence decisions about resident life?
- Is there an active family council?
- Are residents told how to report complaints?
- Can you have a copy of the resident's bill of rights?

- Can the resident's own doctor visit the home?
- Is a resident nurse available 24 hours a day?
- Can the resident choose which hospital they want to use?
- Do the nursing services include; a program to promote bowel and bladder continence; a program to prevent pressure sores; the repositioning of the bed-ridden; disability training; help with self- dressing, feeding and grooming?
- What therapies are available?
- Is there a variety of equipment?
- Does the social worker know the residents?
- What does she or he do?
- Is transportation to hospital, etc., charged as extra?
- Are footcare, eyecare and dentist services available?
- Can personal laundry be done in the home?
- Are hairdressing services available? At extra cost?
- Can small children visit?
- Can residents' pets visit?
- Does the home have pets of its own?
- Are reading materials – books and newspapers – available?
- Is mail delivered throughout the week?
- Can you have a list of things that are charged as extra?
- When you visit the home, what is your impression of the residents?
- How are they dressed?
- Do they seem to be clean? Is there a smell of body odor?
- Do you notice any physical restraints being used?
- What kind of interaction do you see between staff and patients?
- Does any specific cultural group dominate? How will this affect your family?
- How does the home accommodate linguistic and religious needs?
- Does the facility itself seem clean? How is the odor in the building?

- What is your impression of the dining area?
- What is your impression of the activity room?
- Are there activity calendars posted?
- Do the activities on offer interest the prospective resident?
- Are they available at weekends?
- Do the residents appear to enjoy what they are doing?
- Is each resident supplied with a bedside stand, reading light, chest of drawers and comfortable chair?
- Is there enough closet space?
- Is there room to manage a wheelchair?
- Is there a call button near the bed?
- Try to visit the facility at mealtime, and ask yourself if there are enough staff members to help residents eat?
- Does the food smell and look good? Is it served at an appropriate temperature?
- Are residents offered choices?
- Are there water pitchers and glasses on the tables? Are the residents encouraged to drink?
- Are people rushed through their meals or allowed time to eat slowly?
- Is the dining room pleasant?
- Is there conversation between residents during the meal?
- Do they seem to be enjoying their food – do many leave their plates untouched?
- Are the therapy rooms clean?
- What are the rooms like – are they clean, cheerful and well-lit?
- Are bathrooms conveniently located?
- Do they have handgrips near all toilets and baths?
- Are call buttons available in the bathrooms?
- Is the home in good repair?
- Is the temperature acceptable?
- Is the noise level within reasonable limits?

- Are telephones available for private conversation, including for residents in wheelchairs?
- Are rooms, halls and stairs well-lit?
- Are there handrails in all corridors?
- Can you see fire extinguishers and a sprinkler system?
- Does the home have fire drills?
- Is there a system to watch for residents who tend to wander?
- How did the staff behave towards you when they met you?
- Does the administrator seem to know the residents?
- Do staff members know residents by name?
- Do they maintain contact with them when speaking?
- Do they treat them with dignity and respect?
- Is residents' privacy respected?

Working Towards a Better Future

Nursing homes are far from perfect today, and there is every reason to suppose that they will be no better in the foreseeable future. We can work together to change this. How? By demanding a full service, and refusing to tolerate shabby treatment of the nation's elders. By recognizing that, in order to provide properly for those who need most help, we must accept higher tax levels than we might like. By campaigning at local and state level to have public funds spent on the old and the needy instead of less urgent issues. By helping nursing staff secure adequate living wages and good staffing levels. By recognizing the nursing care crisis as the pressing issue it is. By not hiding our heads in the sand and hoping that someone else will take care of things. Public money belongs to us all. We must insist that we have our say on how it's spent, and we can build a better future for tomorrow's elders.